See Again!

See Again!

Reversing and Preventing Macular Degeneration

Alexander M. Eaton, M.D.

Three Rivers Press
New York

The program described in this book is based on the latest research available, and on my own experience with patients in whom I have seen impressive results. Science is constantly coming up with new information, and as we learn more about macular degeneration, modifications may be made to the recommendations in this book. The MD Four-Step Program is intended as a supplement to, not a substitute for, conventional medical therapy. If you are taking medications, or have any type of health problem, talk with your doctor before beginning the MD Four-Step Program. Similarly, do not stop any ongoing medical treatment for macular degeneration, or for any other health problem, without first consulting your doctor.

Although the MD Four-Step Program has helped many people, macular degeneration is a condition which can vary considerably in its severity, and as a result, there can be no guarantee that it will help everybody.

The names of the individuals in the book have been changed to protect their privacy.

Published by Three Rivers Press, 201 East 50th Street, New York, New York 10022. Member of the Crown Publishing Group.

Random House, Inc. New York, Toronto, London, Sydney, Auckland

www.randomhouse.com

Three Rivers Press is a registered trademark of Random House, Inc.

Printed in the United States of America

Design by Rhea Braunstein

Library of Congress Cataloging-in-Publication Data

Eaton, Alexander M.
See again! : reversing and preventing macular degeneration / Alexander M. Eaton. — 1st ed.
p. cm.
1. Retinal degeneration—Popular works. 2. Retinal degeneration—Diet therapy. 3. Antioxidants. I. Title.
RE661.M3E28 1999
617.7'35—dc21 99-12339
CIP

ISBN 0-609-80334-4

10 9 8 7 6 5 4 3 2 1

First Edition

To my patients, from whom I have learned so much.

And to my father, William Mellon Eaton,
who practiced law for 35 years and who encouraged exercise,
good nutrition, and hard work all his life.

CONTENTS

Acknowledgments

Writing a book draws together many people, with many contributions. Consequently, there are many to thank, for without them there would be no book. I would like to thank my parents, William and Elizabeth Eaton, for providing the love, support, and education that enabled me to do this work, and my sisters, Carolyn, Sarah, and Lisa, for giving me the support and encouragement to pursue my goals.

A number of people have helped me with various sections of the book. I am grateful to Myriam Bouchard, O.D., for her assistance and helpful review of the sunglass lens section; to Jeff Singer, M.D., an ophthalmologist in Louisiana, for taking time to review the text for accuracy; to Mary Fox, R.D., L.D., Jamie Gates Galeana, M.S., R.D., L.D., and Ginger Patterson, Ph.D., R.D., L.D., for reviewing my chapters on diet and nutrition; and to Alis Willoughby, C.P.T., a sports trainer, for assistance with the exercise section.

I would also like to thank my publishers, the Crown Publishing Group, and my editor, PJ Dempsey, for believing in this project, directing their energy into every aspect of the book, and making the dream come true. Bob Silverstein, my agent, has been instrumental in helping me shape the book into a user-friendly format.

My special thanks to Marian Betancourt, a superb editor who taught me how a book is structured, organized, and made more interesting to readers.

Ultimately, this entire program would not have been possible without the contributions of my assistant writer, Sue Layton Denham, whose review of my work has made it easier to read for those without a medical background.

Introduction: It's Time to Save Your Sight!

Many people—including some doctors—believe that macular degeneration (MD) is a natural condition of aging, and that there is little we can do to prevent it. This is not true. You do not have to get macular degeneration. Most of its causes are related to lifestyle choices. By eliminating those risk factors with proper nutrition and sun protection, you can live a long life and see clearly.

Though there are effective treatments to prevent visual loss from glaucoma, and restore vision loss due to cataracts, there is no effective treatment to restore vision in the vast majority of people with macular degeneration. Few people know that the retina uses more oxygen than other parts of the body, and thus needs more antioxidants to prevent oxidative stress. The retinal pigment is made of carotenoids that are a natural part of our diet if we eat properly. Our eyes need more zinc, vitamin C, and vitamin E, too, because those nutrients are essential to preventing oxidative stress. The macula need never wear out if we replace the essential components and avoid the oxidative stress that causes wear and tear and, ultimately, aging.

I am writing this book because so many people have come to me with macular degeneration in its advanced stages. This saddens me. I know that if they had taken steps—the steps in my MD Four-Step Program—earlier, they would have prevented it. Fortunately, many others have come to me in time, and although they have already begun to get early age-related macular degeneration, I have been able to help them halt the progress of this disease and in many cases reverse the effects and restore their lives.

The term "age-related macular degeneration" implies that it is an inevitable product of aging, but all we need do is look at my patient Paul to see this is not true. Paul is seventy-two and had been gradually losing his vision. He had worked for the Chevrolet division of General Motors in Michigan for thirty years. He and his wife had worked hard, raised six children, and waited until the youngest boy finished high school before retiring and moving to Florida for what he called a permanent vacation.

Both Paul and his wife enjoy golf, traveling, and reading, and are actively involved in their new community. Yet his gradual decline in vision was threatening to end his ability to do the things he enjoyed. When Paul first came to see me, his vision had deteriorated to 20/60, and he was having difficulty reading and driving. When I examined him I found his macula—the central portion of his retina, responsible for his central vision—was deteriorating.

I started Paul on the MD Four-Step Program of vitamins, diet, exercise, and sun protection. After a year his vision improved to 20/30. He is now able to read and drive without difficulty, and he is no longer worried about losing his independence. Happily, he is able to enjoy the lifestyle that brought him to Florida in the first place.

My patients are the lucky ones. The experience for millions of Americans, after years of visits to the eye doctor, is that little has been done and their vision has deteriorated. They have progressed from glasses to a magnifier, then to the services of a low-vision specialist. Eventually they cannot read at all and progress to audio books. During all this time, the doctor has continued to say there is nothing more to be done. Or is there?

Macular degeneration has been called the leading cause of irreversible vision loss in the United States, Western Europe, and most industrialized nations. ABC-TV's newsmagazine program *20/20* called it "the epidemic of the twenty-first century." It is estimated that more than 15 million people in the United States have the condition and that it will someday affect 30 million baby boomers. One in three Americans over the age of seventy-five can expect to be diagnosed with the disease.

Your future is not that grim. *You do not have to get macular degeneration.* A wealth of evidence shows that this disorder is not a normal, inevitable part of the aging process. Though it is true that macular degeneration occurs more frequently and severely in mature adults, it is more likely a result of lifelong, cumulative exposure to oxidative stress, vascular disease, and sunlight than to simple aging.

Many factors are within your control to mitigate retinal damage. The baby boomers, who are becoming our senior citizens, have never been known to resignedly accept the status quo. If you are reading this book, you probably feel the same way.

Science is accumulating a wealth of knowledge about how lifestyle changes can improve our health and well-being. We hear frequently, for example, about the importance of diet and lifestyle to cardiovascular health; it is time to learn what we can do to save our vision. It is time to take control of our visual health.

Part 1 of this book will help you understand how your eyes work, how macular degeneration develops, and how the MD Four-Step Program will prevent that development. I will show you how nutrition and your vision are linked, and how your eye responds to all kinds of light, including reflected light.

Part 2 gives you the information you need to begin my MD Four-Step Program. There are vitamin supplement requirements, food tables prepared by professional nutritionists, and information about keeping those nutrients in your foods through proper selection, storage, and preparation.

There are chapters on eliminating lifestyle risk like smoking and lack of exercise, and a very big chapter to help you select the proper sunglasses to protect your eyes from the particular light rays implicated in macular degeneration. Part 3 contains recipes from well-known gourmet chefs to help you enjoy meals with the nutrients you need to prevent macular degeneration.

The appendices provide my own test results on scores of different types of sunglasses as well as discussion of some of the popular brands. There is also information you need if you are planning to get prescription sunglasses.

Hardly a day goes by that I do not see a new patient who is losing vision from macular degeneration. Typically, these people tell me they know they have macular degeneration but they have been told there is nothing that can be done about it. My desire to change those perceptions, and to share the growing body of evidence that there is indeed much we can do for macular degeneration, formed the basis of the MD Four-Step Program, and motivated me to write this book.

Here's to your good visual health!

PART I

THE NATURAL HISTORY OF YOUR EYES

1

Understanding How Your Eyes Work

Before we explore our options, it is important that you learn more about how your eyes work, how macular degeneration develops, and how risk factors make you vulnerable. Macular degeneration is a disease with many different forms that can affect our vision to varying degrees. The most common forms tend to be mild, and to have only a minimal effect on vision. Eventually, however, all forms of MD, even the milder ones, can lead to the loss of central vision.

Until recently, doctors have thought little could be done to prevent the onset of macular degeneration. Treatment has been limited to surgical intervention in the most serious form of the disease, which is present in only 10 to 15 percent of cases. Rather than simply waiting and watching for signs of the only surgically treatable form, a growing number of doctors are actually taking action to prevent the development of macular degeneration. We are reporting excellent results from a combination of vitamin supplements, diet, exercise, and sun protection to slow and actually prevent the progression of the disease.

Although extensive evidence from around the world shows that this approach works, it has been largely ignored by the American medical community. But this is beginning to change. We are on the verge of a major revolution in the treatment of macular degeneration.

But, you may ask, can I act on this information if it is not widely accepted in the general medical community? If it's that good, shouldn't I have heard more about it? Not necessarily. The medical community has always been slow to accept change. The evolution of cataract surgery is a good example. Less than ten years ago, almost all cataract surgery involved sutures. Then a few progressive surgeons found it could be done without sutures. The response from the general medical community was to criticize the technique, claiming it to be unsafe, even reckless. Today it is well recognized that the sutureless technique is safer, faster, and better overall, and most cataract surgery is now performed that way.

The same is true for this revolutionary approach to preserving vision. Doctors throughout the United States are beginning to acknowledge the merits of nutritional supplements, proper diet, regular exercise, and sun protection, and more will follow. It is time for a change, and for people to know there is something they can do to improve their visual health.

The MD Four-Step Program

I developed the MD Four-Step Program for my patients, and have prescribed it for years. It is both revolutionary and simple—revolutionary because it challenges the long-held belief that the onset and progression of macular degeneration are inevitable as we age, and simple because the four steps are within reach of anyone who is motivated to achieve better vision. These steps are as follows:

1. Begin a program of antioxidant supplements to reduce your risk of oxidative stress.

2. Increase your dietary intake of antioxidants, vitamins, and minerals, and reduce the amount of fat you eat.
3. Eliminate lifestyle risk factors such as smoking and heavy drinking. Begin a regular exercise program.
4. Protect your eyes with a hat and sunglasses that will screen out ultraviolet and blue light. But first, let's take a look at how your eyes work, and how they become vulnerable to macular degeneration.

The Anatomy of the Eye

The eye is a sphere the size of a quarter, which rests in an opening in your skull. For such a small organ, it is one of the busiest parts of your body. It needs more oxygen, zinc, and antioxidants than do much larger organs like your heart, brain, and lungs. When light enters your eyes, a complex set of reactions takes place so that you can see.

The eye is made of layers (figure 1.1) called *tunics.* The curved, fibrous layer helps maintain the shape of the eye and is composed of the transparent cornea and the opaque white sclera. The middle, vascular tunic contains the colored iris with the dark pupil at its center, the ciliary body (muscle and ligaments), and the choroid, which contains blood vessels. The third, innermost layer is the retina.

There are two compartments in the eye: the anterior chamber in the front, and the vitreous cavity in the middle and back of the eye. The anterior chamber is filled with a fluid called aqueous humor, which is produced by the ciliary body and provides oxygen, glucose, and proteins to the cornea, iris, and lens. The aqueous humor is responsible for maintaining the internal pressure and shape of the eye. The vitreous body, a clear substance like egg white, fills the remaining 80 percent of the eye, the middle and back. (This substance is actually a matrix of collagen fibers [protein], which is what gives Jell-O its characteristic consistency.)

Light enters your eye through the cornea and passes

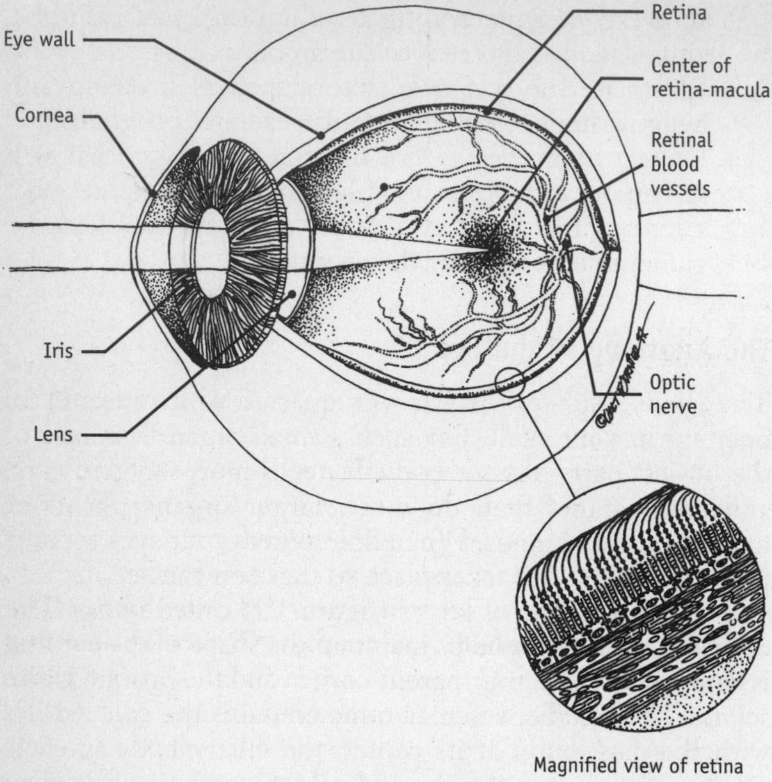

Figure 1.1. The Eye.

through the pupil in the iris. The iris, like a camera shutter, constricts in bright light to reduce the amount of light that can enter. In a darker place, it dilates to allow more light in.

Your eyes focus like a camera, too. The ability of the eyes to focus on an object nearby is called accommodation. Ciliary muscles in the eye respond automatically to the closeness or distance of an object by altering the shape of the lens. This changes the angle of incoming light rays and allows for their focus on the retina. As the body ages, the elasticity of the lens decreases, as does the speed and power of accommodation. This is known as presbyopia (see page 9).

Wherever you direct your gaze, the image is focused by the front of your eye onto the retina, a complex layer of cells at the back of your eye that convert it into a signal. The signal is then passed by your optic nerve to the brain, where it is converted back into the image you actually see. This process is not unlike using a video camera. When we aim a video camera, the lens system captures images that are then converted into electronic impulses, which are transmitted via cable to a television set, where they are converted back into images for viewing.

However, there is one big difference. With a video camera the entire image is clear. With human vision, sharp focus is restricted to the central part of the image. Try to read a book while holding it off to the side and looking straight ahead. While you may be able to decipher the title, it is impossible to read regular-size print.

The eye, then, is designed to provide us with sharp vision in the center of our viewing world, and the central portion of the retina—responsible for this fine vision—is called the macula. When this is damaged, we lose our ability to focus precisely, and images become blurred. Peripheral (side) vision remains intact, which helps with normal activities such as walking.

The ophthalmic artery and its branches supply the eye with blood. Fat and lipids can clog these arteries just like the arteries in your heart. Hypertension affects them, too. When blood vessels of the eye malfunction, they can contribute to the development of macular degeneration.

Your eye needs lots of oxygen. Because so much light comes through and interacts with the oxygen, there is lots of stress, too. There are two types of oxygen inside your eye. Stable oxygen is necessary to sustain vision. Unstable oxygen (in the form of free radicals) is unwanted and results in tissue damage. The body produces free-radical "scavengers" to eliminate excess free radicals and prevent damage to your eye. Trouble starts when free radicals exceed scavengers, and thus are not eliminated. Unchecked, these excess free radicals injure your eye, and visual loss may be the result. This damage is called oxidative stress.

Sunlight, smoking, pollution, and contaminants in your food can all produce excess free radicals that damage your eye, particularly the lens and the retina. When the lens becomes damaged, it can lead to the development of a cataract, and a reduction in vision. When the retina becomes damaged, it can lead to the development of macular degeneration.

Common Conditions of the Eye

Nearsightedness, also known as myopia, occurs when the eye's lens focuses an image in front of the retina rather than directly on it, because the eyeball is usually longer than normal from front to back, which makes objects at a distance hard to see clearly. The condition starts in childhood and gets worse until it generally stabilizes around the age of thirty. Because most myopic people wear corrective lenses, which provide some protection for their eyes, they are less likely to develop macular degeneration. Also, people who wear glasses are more inclined to wear sunglasses than those who are not used to having glasses on their faces. The slightly smaller risk of a myopic child developing macular degeneration later in life is offset, however, by the increased risk of glaucoma.

Farsightedness—hyperopia—means that only distant objects are seen clearly, because the lens focuses the image behind the retina rather than on it. This usually occurs because the eyeball is shorter than normal from front to back. Your eyes can accommodate to overcome this error until you get older. As we age, however, our ability to accommodate is gradually lost, so we need glasses to correct this condition. Farsighted people are more prone to macular degeneration.

Astigmatism occurs when your cornea is shaped like a football rather than a basketball. The refracting power of your eye is not equal all around, and the result is blurred vision. In most people, glasses, contact lenses, or surgery can overcome the effects on vision.

Color blindness may be either congenital or acquired. Our ability to see color is created by the way our retina absorbs light from short, middle, or long wavelengths (see chapter 5). The most common congenital defect is red-green distortion, in which affected individuals confuse reds, browns, olives, and golds. It affects both eyes in about 8 percent of men and fewer than 1 percent of women—or about 5 percent of the population in this country.

Conditions of the Aging Eye

A host of other conditions and circumstances can affect your eyes as you get older; that is why annual eye examinations are so important from age forty on, not just to correct vision but to watch for the development of any degenerative conditions such as glaucoma, cataracts, and macular degeneration. See your doctor immediately, of course, should you have any loss or change in your vision. By delaying treatment, you could end up with irreversible vision loss that might have been prevented.

Presbyopia is the gradual loss of the eye's ability to accommodate for focusing on near objects. By the age of forty, most of us begin to need reading glasses to see the small print in newspapers and on labels. This does not mean we are developing any of the other conditions of the aging eye, such as glaucoma, cataracts, or macular degeneration.

Glaucoma is like high blood pressure of the eye. The pressure is caused by the buildup of aqueous humor, which normally drains away as fast as it is secreted. This buildup can be the result of a faulty drainage channel between the back of the cornea and the iris. Drug treatment usually helps lower the pressure, and laser surgery can open a blocked channel or create one if needed. Untreated, glaucoma can cause blindness. Glaucoma is the leading cause of blindness in African Americans, and the third leading cause of blindness in white Americans. The opposite is true of macular degeneration, which is more common in whites. Other risk factors for glaucoma are severe myopia, genetic predisposition, and vascular diseases such as diabetes. Glaucoma typically causes loss of peripheral vision—the opposite of macular degeneration, in which one loses central vision.

Cataracts are a clouding of the lens in the eye, which reduces or blurs the light entering the eye. It is most common as a condition of aging or as a result of inflammation or trauma to the eye. It can also be congenital, but this is rare. Cataracts typically begin to develop around forty to fifty years of age, and progress slowly over time. They are usually detected during a routine examination. Surgery to remove the cloudy lens and replace it with a clear implant has advanced over the last ten to twenty years, to a point where this operation is now very safe and effective in the hands of a skilled ophthalmic surgeon. An incision is made in the cornea and the opaque lens is removed. An artificial lens is then inserted and fixed in place by means of plastic loops.

Macular degeneration is the gradual loss of central vision because of degeneration of the central portion of the retina. This condition can be prevented with my MD Four-Step Program, and is what this book is all about.

Diagnosing the Condition of the Eye

To properly diagnose the condition of your eye, we need to know not only what symptoms or vision problem brought you to the doctor, but also a general description of your past and present health, your lifestyle, and your family health history. Then your eyes are tested in several ways. If you have been getting routine eye examinations all your life, you are probably familiar with these tests.

Visual acuity. We have all had to read that chart with the big *E* on top. This is the Snellen chart, designed to test how far you can see. The big *E* represents vision of 20/400. If you cannot read that big *E*, you are legally blind. If you can see at 20/40, it means you can see an object at twenty feet that a person with normal vision can see at forty feet. Normal vision is 20/20. In Europe this is measured in meters, so 6/6 is normal vision.

Pupils are examined for abnormalities in your retina and your optic nerve, such as low blood flow, inflammation, trauma, tumors, or any congenital abnormalities.

Extraocular alignment and motility. The alignment of your eyes is tested to see if you are cross-eyed, a condition known as strabismus, or if there is a problem with the muscles and nerves that move your eyes. Impairment of the motility of the eye can occur in both children and adults, and tends to arise from such conditions as diabetes, thyroid disease, trauma, tumors, and immune disorders.

Confrontation visual field is a test for peripheral vision. Problems in your visual field could occur as a result of glaucoma, optic nerve disease, retinal disorders, impaired blood flow, and central nervous system disorders such as a tumor or stroke.

Intraocular pressure test. This test is done with a puff of air, or with a device that presses on the cornea. You can have high pressure in your eye without knowing it. When the pressure is very high, it can cause pain, headaches, nausea, and glaucoma.

Slit lamp exam. The slit lamp is a microscope mounted on a table with a beam of light that allows examination of both the front of your eye and your retina under very high magnification. This test can detect early signs of macular degeneration.

Indirect ophthalmoscopy is used to detect retinal tears, detachments, tumors, and other retinal problems.

Now that you have a better idea how your eyes work, let's take a look at how macular degeneration develops.

2

How Macular Degeneration Develops

When Dr. Emma Williams retired from her job in Indiana as a university professor, she moved to Florida so she could write and paint and play tennis. She had already been diagnosed with the beginnings of macular degeneration in her right eye, but had not been given any information about the condition other than that she would need to rely more on her peripheral vision in that eye.

After she moved to Florida, Dr. Williams was driving from Orlando one Friday afternoon when suddenly her left eye began to itch, and when she lifted her hand to rub her eye, she found she could not see out of her right eye. Before she allowed herself to panic, she went to see the doctor from whom she had been getting glasses. He referred her to a retina specialist. When she arrived at the specialist's office, she was given a cursory examination, after which the doctor told her she had developed a serious form of macular degeneration that causes the blood vessels in the retina to bleed. She was told to come back Monday, when laser surgery would be performed to stop the bleeding. They couldn't do anything until then. The doctor told her there was not much effective treatment for her condition, and she would eventually go blind. Dr. Williams felt her hopes for her future dashed, and wondered if she would spend the rest of her life in darkness with a white cane.

But Dr. Williams was a smart woman who knew how to do research. She resented being treated so coldly and brushed off by the doctors. She was not blind to the treatment she was getting. After two more doctors gave her the same bad news, she came to me. I was able to halt the progress of her macular degeneration and put her on my MD Four-Step Program. Dr. Williams has continued her writing, painting, and tennis.

What my patient went through is all too common, because so many doctors don't take the time to educate their patients, and often they are skeptical about the latest research, or they simply have not kept up with it.

The Layers of the Retina

Your retina is like the film in your camera. And like film, it needs to be properly cared for or your vision will be fuzzy or blurry. If you open your camera and expose it to too much light, the film will be destroyed and there will be no picture at all. Failure to protect your retina from excess light will result in similar damage.

Your retina is made of layers of cells, nerve fibers, and blood vessels, which all have a role in keeping your vision intact. Here's what you need to know about the parts of your retina, its supporting structures, and how they are affected by macular degeneration (see figure 2.1).

Retinal pigment epithelium (RPE) is a layer of cells beneath the photoreceptors and on top of the choroid and Bruch's membrane, upon which the photoreceptors depend for nourishment. This is like the topsoil in your garden. Common to all forms of macular degeneration is some type of problem with your RPE.

Photoreceptors are neural cells located on top of the RPE layer that convert light into a signal, and they lead a very active life! Think of them as pushy little paparazzi,

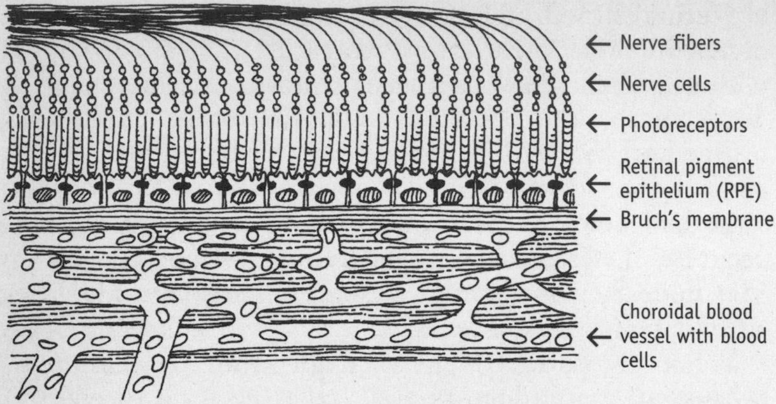

Figure 2.1. A Healthy Retina

each taking up to sixty pictures a second, that let you see the world around you. All this earnest activity results in the accumulation of waste (all those empty film cartons!). Photoreceptors are constantly being replaced, with the help of the RPE. It is not surprising, then, that over time the RPE can wear out from all this activity, and cell by-products called drusen accumulate on Bruch's membrane (see below). Photoreceptors contain high concentrations of polyunsaturated fats as well as a protein called rhodopsin, which contains vitamin A. The RPE helps obtain fresh supplies of vitamin A from our blood supply as it is needed and delivers it to the photoreceptors.

Rods and cones are the two photoreceptor cell types found in the retina that convert an image to a signal. Each eye has about six million cones and 120 million rods. Cones are responsible for fine detailed vision, central vision, and color vision in brightly lit environments. Rods are responsible for night vision and peripheral vision.

Nerve cell and fiber layers are present on top of the photoreceptors. They transmit the signal from the photoreceptors to the optic nerve, and on to the brain, where it is converted back into an image.

Retinal blood vessels are located within the nerve cell layers on top of the photoreceptors and provide them with nutrients. They have tight junctions and therefore do not leak.

Retinal glial cells provide structural support within the retina.

Bruch's membrane is another layer, a collagen film that separates the RPE and the choroid. The drusen (see above) that build up like sludge on Bruch's membrane will, over time, damage the RPE and photoreceptors and cause visual loss, but it is usually not until we reach fifty years of age or older that the damage is sufficient to result in visual impairment. Therefore, the sooner the damage is prevented or reduced, the lower our risk of vision loss. In some cases the weakened Bruch's membrane is no longer able to resist the growth of choroidal blood vessels, and this results in the development of "wet" macular degeneration (see page 17).

Choroid is the layer of blood vessels, pigment, and connective tissue that rests under Bruch's membrane and nourishes the RPE. Blood drains from the choroid through the four veins equally spaced around the equator of the eye. The RPE serves as the barrier between the choroidal blood vessels, which do not have tight junctions and therefore leak, and the retina. When abnormal blood vessels grow under the retina as a result of wet age-related macular degeneration, they also leak. This is because they typically arise from the choroidal blood vessels.

Macula is defined in two ways. It is typically used in this book, and by most people, to mean the 5.5-mm central portion of the retina, the center of which has a slightly darker color than the surrounding tissue. This area is composed of nerve fibers and cells, retinal blood vessels, photoreceptors, RPE, the choroid, and the choroidal blood vessels—all the tissue layers responsible for central vision. It is also defined anatomically by scientists as the posterior retina, which contains yellow pigment (xanthophyll); it is the macula, at the center of the retina, which is damaged by macular degeneration.

Macula pigment has two parts. The pigment called xanthophyll, in the nerve cell layer (see above), and the pigment underneath the photoreceptors, in the RPE and the choroid, known as melanin. Both types of pigment help to filter out and absorb the blue and visible light implicated in the development of macular degeneration.

Types of Macular Degeneration (MD)

There are three types of macular degeneration. In the vast majority of cases, it begins as what we call the "dry" form. Typically, after a number of years, it can progress to the "wet" form, or to the third type, a pigment epithelial detachment (PED). It is rare to see wet macular degeneration or a pigment epithelial detachment without evidence of preexisting dry macular degeneration. Macular degeneration is typically referred to as age-related macular degeneration (AMD or ARMD), because it occurs almost exclusively in the senior population.

Dry MD

The most common form of MD, this accounts for 85 percent of all cases. For the majority of people, this is the first form of MD to develop. It tends to be mild in the early stages, and only with the passage of many years does it lead to a severe reduction in vision. Because this type shows no fluid, blood, or protein leakage between retinal layers, it is called "dry" MD.

Geographic atrophy. This type of dry MD is characterized by the absence of RPE cells, which results in photoreceptor death and visual loss (figure 2.2). Typically, with this condition, blood flow to the choroidal blood vessels below the area of cell loss is also reduced.

Drusen are round, slightly elevated protein deposits resulting from damage to the macula (figure 2.3). They are

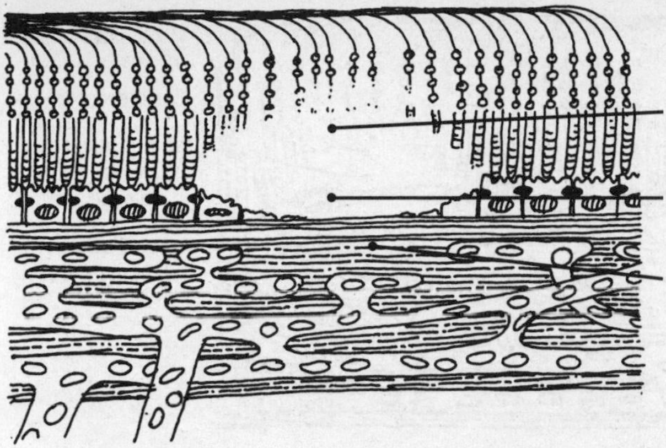

Figure 2.2. Dry Macular Degeneration—Geographic Atrophy. Retinal pigment epithelial cell loss results in photoreceptor loss and decreased vision.

one of the earliest indicators of MD, and can be detected with the slit lamp. Drusen can be hard or soft, and sometimes they also develop in the peripheral retina. This damage occurs even before there is any noticeable effect on your vision. Over time they damage the RPE and cause photoreceptor death and visual loss. The presence of large, thick drusen also increases the risk of developing wet macular degeneration.

Wet MD

A less common but more severe form of macular degeneration occurs when choroidal blood vessels grow through Bruch's membrane and directly under the RPE, the photoreceptors, or both. Once the blood vessels grow through Bruch's membrane, they expand quickly, causing damage to the RPE and the photoreceptors, which leads to rapid vision loss. Blood vessels are not meant to be in this space, and when they get there they cause trouble (figures 2.3 and 2.4). Choroidal neovascularization (CNV) is the medical term for wet MD; the condition gets its name from the

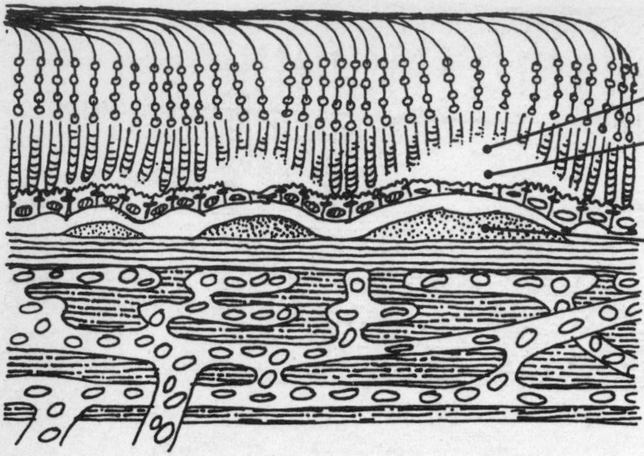

Figure 2.3. Dry Macular Degeneration—Drusen.
Accumulation of cell by-products called drusen results in photoreceptor loss and decreased vision.

leakage of fluid, blood, and protein from these abnormal blood vessels. If the condition is caught early, laser treatment can stop the growth of blood vessels, prevent further vision loss, and even, in some rare cases, improve vision.

Pigment Epithelial Detachment (PED)

This is the least common form of macular degeneration, typically resulting in severe vision loss. It is caused by the formation of a blister of fluid leaking through Bruch's membrane from the blood vessels below, elevating the retina like a bump under a carpet. In some cases, immediate treatment can prevent severe vision loss.

Symptoms of Macular Degeneration

You cannot feel any degeneration happening in your macula, but you may notice changes in your vision, such as difficulty reading the newspaper or seeing road signs. Nothing to be concerned about, you think—must be time for new glasses. Then you notice that letters are missing in the middle of the page. You can't remember this happening

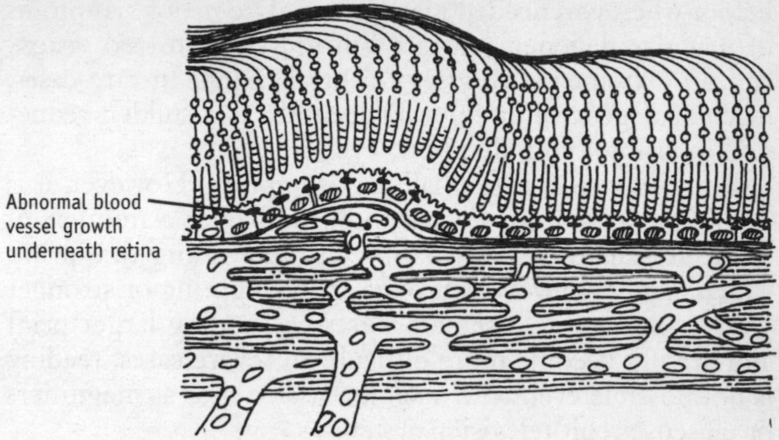

Figure 2.4. Wet Macular Degeneration—Early Stage.
Day 1: Early growth of blood vessels underneath the retina disrupts retinal pigment ephithelial cells and photoreceptors, and results in visual distortion.

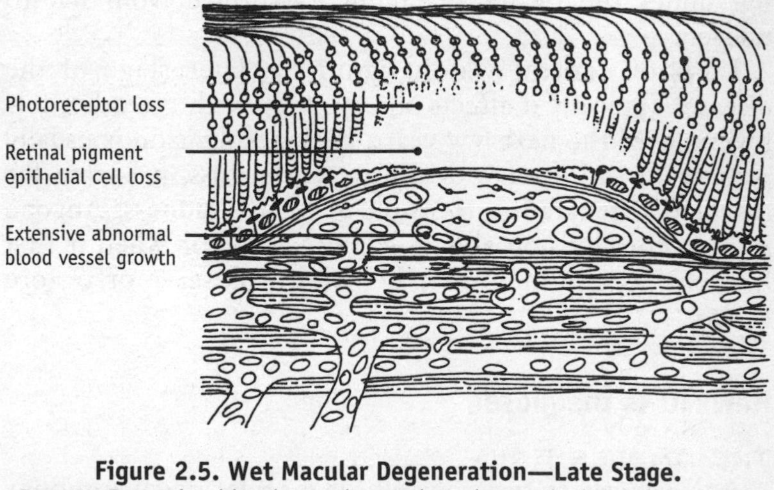

Figure 2.5. Wet Macular Degeneration—Late Stage.
Day 14: Extensive blood vessel growth underneath the retina results in retinal pigment epithelial cell loss, and subsequent photoreceptor loss and decreased vision.

before when you needed new glasses. The major symptoms of macular degeneration are blurred or distorted vision, and, in extreme cases, loss of central vision. In rare cases, macular degeneration appears abruptly as a sudden reduction in vision, typically in one eye.

Blurred vision is the hallmark symptom. However, it is a mildly blurred vision that intensifies over a number of years. It usually begins as difficulty in reading fine print, which can be improved through better lighting or stronger glasses. But as the disease progresses, reading larger print and driving become more difficult. In severe cases, reading is not possible even with such low-vision aids as magnifiers or closed-circuit television systems.

Distortion, also known as metamorphopsia, is most noticeable when we look at linear objects such as vertical blinds or light poles. An object that appears wavy or crooked is a warning sign of wet macular degeneration, the most serious form of the disease, and it signals the need for an eye exam within twenty-four to forty-eight hours. Distortion is typically caused by abnormal blood vessels growing under the retina, changing its surface from flat to uneven.

Loss of central vision signifies a later stage of the disease. Typically it affects one eye first, with the other following over the next few years. Peripheral vision is usually preserved, and even with central vision loss, it is rare for macular degeneration to result in total blindness. Anyone losing central vision should contact a doctor when it first happens, as treatment may be able to preserve or restore vision.

How MD Is Diagnosed

The Amsler Grid

An easy way to test yourself for macular degeneration is with a widely used device called an Amsler grid, which uses

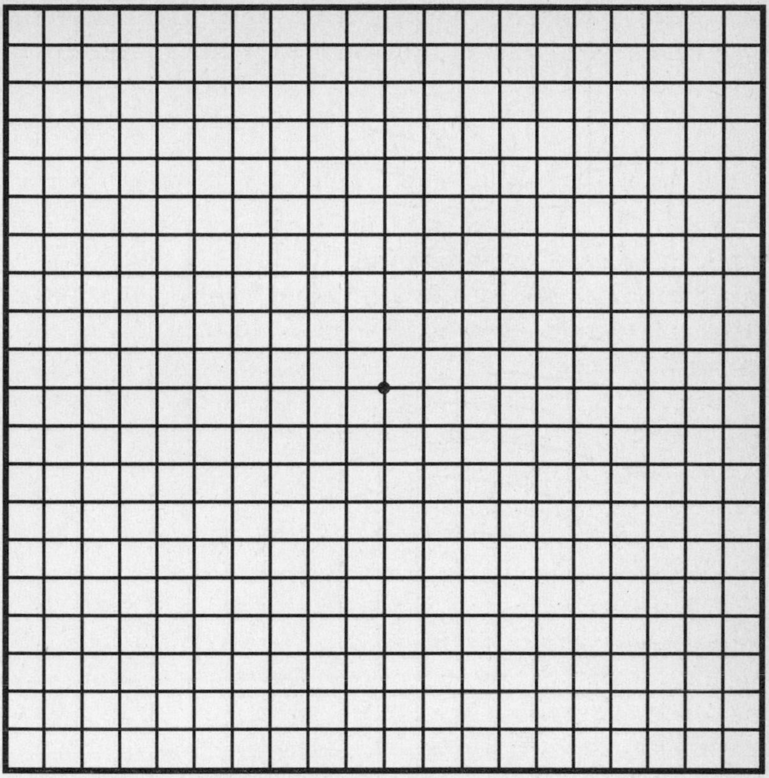

Figure 2.6. An Amsler Grid

distortion as a means of monitoring for the onset of wet macular degeneration. The ruled grid, named for the physician who developed it, has a black or white dot in the center (figure 2.6). With one eye covered, focus on the central dot. If the ruled lines appear distorted or wavy (figure 2.7), or if there are dark spots or missing areas in the grid, it could be an early sign of wet macular degeneration. Call a doctor immediately if this happens. Prompt treatment may mean the difference between preserving reading vision and losing it. Doctors frequently use the Amsler grid to detect wet MD before it causes severe vision loss.

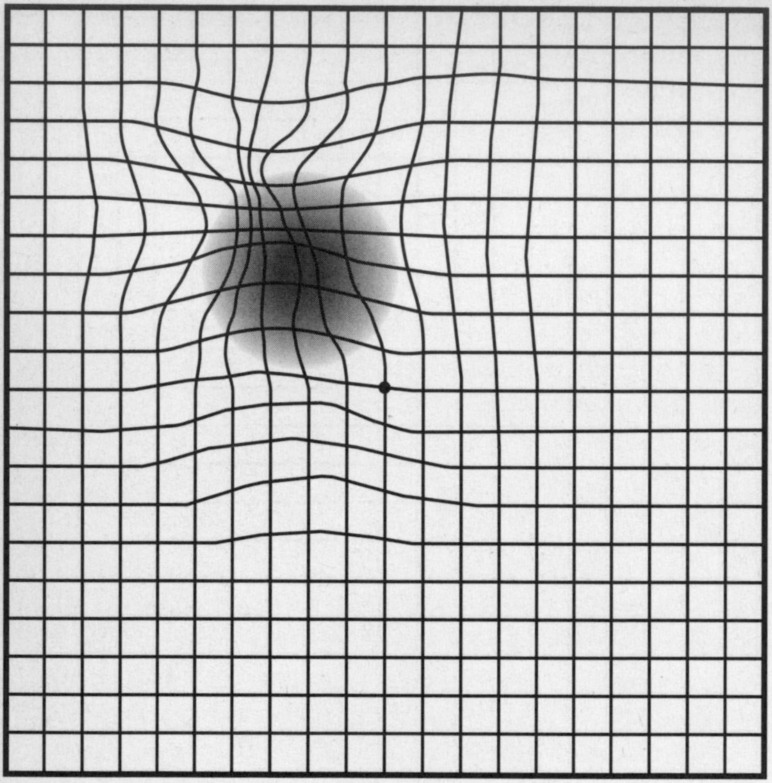

Figure 2.7. How an Amsler Grid might appear to a person with wet macular degeneration.

Slit Lamp Exam

Macular degeneration can be diagnosed by looking into the retina through a device called a slit lamp, which will reveal areas of drusen in dry macular degeneration. If you have wet MD, the telltale sign is fluid, either clear or bloody, which causes an elevation of the retina and the RPE. If there are signs of wet MD, a fluorescein angiogram (FA) is called for.

Fluorescein Angiography (FA)

The fluorescein angiogram shows where the blood vessels are, and serves as a road map for treatment. It also helps to define changes in the macula and identify areas of cell loss and damage, which can help explain why vision has deteriorated.

This test is usually done in the doctor's office by sitting you in front of a large camera system designed to take pictures of the inside of your eye. The camera is about two feet high and secured to a table. Photos of your retina are taken, then a dye called sodium fluorescein is injected into your arm. The dye travels through your bloodstream to the blood vessels of the retina. Fluorescein absorbs light of one color and emits it in another color, which, in combination with the right filters, helps us see. Compared against the pre-injection photograph of the eye, a fluorescein angiogram provides a more detailed view of the retinal blood vessels, their integrity, and the integrity of the RPE cell layer upon which the photoreceptors are located.

Remember, there are two layers of blood vessels in your eye: the retinal blood vessels, which have tight junctions, and the choroidal blood vessels, which do not. The RPE serves as the barrier between the choroidal blood supply and the retina. When abnormal blood vessels grow (CNV), they do not have tight junctions and they leak because they arise from the choroidal blood supply. The FA helps us see this.

Fluorescein angiography is a relatively safe test. The dye does not contain iodine, as do many of the dyes used for X-ray and other radiologic studies. Side effects from the angiogram may include nausea in about 5 percent of people, but this passes within a few minutes. Hives, itching, and vomiting occur in less than one percent, and even more rare are shock or cardiac arrest.

It used to take a few hours to process the pictures, but with today's high-tech computers we can process the images and print them in a few minutes, so you don't have to wait around for a long time to hear the diagnosis.

Indocyanine Green (ICG)

Another type of angiogram, called an indocyanine green angiogram, is better able to see through blood and to define blood vessel growth that may not be clear with FA. Unless the lesions are clearly defined, laser treatment cannot be done. By using ICG we are able to clearly define lesions, and therefore treat 40 percent of people whose lesions were poorly defined using fluorescein angiography.

This test was used first in 1986, but did not become widely used until the 1990s. Unlike the FA, this dye has iodine, and if you have an allergic reaction to shellfish, you would likely react to this dye, too. You cannot have this test if you have kidney or liver disease, either.

Traditional Treatment for Wet MD

Prevention is the best treatment for MD, and here's why: There is no cure for dry macular degeneration, and laser treatment for wet MD can only reduce further risk of visual loss; it does not restore vision. Early detection and treatment result in the best outcome with laser treatment, but recurrence rates are high, with more than 50 percent of people developing new blood vessel growth and further visual loss within three years of the laser treatment. All we can do with conventional treatment is to prevent it from getting worse.

Laser treatment with a retinal specialist can be done in the doctor's office in five to fifteen minutes, while you are sitting in a chair in front of a specialized slit lamp. A fiber-optic system delivers the laser energy from an adjacent laser source, which looks like a floor-standing personal computer next to the slit lamp. An anesthetic eye drop—similar to the Novocain your dentist uses—subdues any pain in the eye. A contact lens is then placed on your eye to neutralize the effect on the cornea and the lens, and provides a clear view of the retina and the macula.

A picture of the area to be treated—an FA or ICG—is

enlarged and used as a guideline, or map, for the treatment. The laser is then applied to the abnormal blood vessels. Multiple pulses of laser energy pass through the cornea and lens in the same way light passes through the eye. Laser energy is high-energy light that is absorbed by the RPE and the blood in the vessels and turns to heat. This causes them to congeal or harden as egg white hardens when you cook it. This coagulation stops the blood flow in the abnormal blood vessels and prevents further growth, but the retina overlying the blood vessels and immediately adjacent to them is irreversibly damaged. It becomes scar tissue.

After the laser treatment you go home. You need to refrain from heavy straining or lifting for a week. Follow-up visits are necessary every few weeks for the first three months, and then every three to six months, to watch the eye for the growth of new abnormal blood vessels. You will need to have additional FA tests on follow-up visits to check the eye for recurrences. If they are caught early, more laser treatment can prevent further vision loss.

New and Experimental Treatments

Although no treatment is now available for the geographic atrophy type of dry MD, current research is looking at treatment with fetal-cell transplants and gene therapy. For people with dry MD and drusen, there is evidence that laser treatment and ReoTherapy, a technique for filtering certain proteins from the blood, can help facilitate the absorption of soft drusen and improve or stabilize vision. In 1999, I will be participating as one of five United States study sites in an FDA study evaluating the efficacy of ReoTherapy for the treatment of people with soft drusen. There is no treatment for hard drusen.

A large prevention trial is under way in the United States to determine precisely the benefits of laser treatment for soft drusen in people with no history of wet MD. In addition to some improvement in vision, there is hope that the laser treatment will reduce the risk of wet MD developing. The study is called the Complications of AMD Prevention Trial (CAPT) and is funded by the National Institutes of Health. We anticipate results around 2004.

Subretinal surgery. Theoretically, surgical removal from under the retina of the blood vessels responsible for wet MD has the potential for less damage to the retina than laser surgery. With less damage, presumably the vision would be better. We call this subretinal surgery. It was first done by Dr. Eugene deJuan and Dr. Robert Machemer at Duke University in the mid-1980s.

I had the good fortune to be at Duke when this work was going on, and to train with Dr. Machemer, who invented the technique we now use to remove the vitreous gel from the eye as well. He used to experiment in his garage in Miami in the early 1970s, trying to remove the white of an egg without cracking the shell (egg white is very similar in consistency to the vitreous gel). He eventually found that by putting a plastic sleeve or tube around a drill bit, he could remove the egg white without cracking the shell. This led to the first "vitreous cutter," which comprised essentially a drill bit, a motor, a tube to remove the fluid, and another tube to replace it. It took time to perfect, but he did it, and now we can remove the vitreous gel with little risk to the eye. The instruments have evolved to the point where many of the ones now used in this surgery are small enough to fit through the eye of a needle.

Before this development, the cornea had to be removed from the eye, and the vitreous gel was extracted by dipping a sponge into it, then pulling out what you could and cutting the strands with a pair of scissors. The technique was crude, and resulted in a high rate of complications.

Despite these wonderful advances in our ability to remove the vitreous gel and the theoretical advantages of subretinal surgery, vision has not improved in most people following surgery. To determine precisely the benefits of subretinal surgery, if any, over such other forms of treatment as laser surgery or no treatment at all, the National Eye Institute (NEI), a division of the National Institutes of Health, has funded a study called the Submacular Surgery Trial (SST). The study will look at the benefits and risks of this type of surgery for the removal of subfoveal choroidal neovascularization (wet macular degeneration). The study began in August 1998, and it will most likely be a few years before the results are known.

Submacular surgery with retinal rotation. It is thought the reason most people do not get visual improvement following subretinal surgery is because the RPE is removed with the blood vessels from under the retina. Without the RPE the retina is not able to survive, and vision is lost. Retinal rotation, in which the retina is slid around so that at the end of the operation it is resting on a healthy layer of RPE cells, is the answer to this problem. Using this technique, it is possible to restore vision in some patients with wet MD.

However, this surgery is very labor-intensive. When I assisted Dr. Machemer during one of the first surgeries of this type, it took nearly eight hours, but the patient achieved significant visual improvement. Recently, a modified technique called a *retinal translocation* has been developed by Dr. deJuan at Johns Hopkins that is significantly faster and safer than the earlier method. While this new technique holds great promise for the small group of patients who qualify, it is still associated with a higher risk of complications than with conventional laser treatment. After a successful operation, it also takes up to a year to adapt to vision that is on an angle (rotated) in one eye and straight in the other. As you can imagine, such simple tasks as walking and keeping one's balance are more difficult for the first few months. All these factors must be considered when deciding on the best treatment for each individual. While these techniques hold great promise in the small group of patients who qualify for the surgery, they are associated with a higher risk of complications than conventional laser treatment. This must be considered in any decision.

Photodynamic therapy (PDT). Now being tested on some patients with wet MD, this is a therapy in which a light-sensitive drug is injected into a vein in the arm, and a low-intensity laser light activates the drug at the disease site in the eye. This results in less injury to adjacent tissues than does treatment with the higher-powered lasers used for conventional laser treatment. Early results are encouraging and show visual improvement in some people with wet MD who would have lost vision if conventional laser treatment had been performed. It looks as though PDT offers advantages over other forms of treatment for wet MD, but as of this writing we are still waiting for the U.S. Food and Drug Administration approval for this treatment. It is anticipated that if there are no surprises in the ongoing study, PDT will be approved by the FDA at the turn of the century.

Thalidomide. This drug was used as a sedative in the late 1950s but was taken off the market when it was found to cause devastating birth defects. Thalidomide interferes with normal blood vessel development, which is why the birth defects occurred. Because wet MD involves growth of abnormal blood vessels, it seems logical to consider using it to prevent and arrest the development of wet MD—at least for people who are not planning to have children. An FDA study has been under way since 1995, the MD Thalidomide Trial, to see if it is beneficial as a treatment.

Antioxidant Therapy. This therapy shows great promise, and I have seen wonderful results with it. Mainstream ophthalmologists, along with the National Eye Institute (NEI), agree that there is now enough evidence that antioxidants may be beneficial to initiate a randomized, controlled study to determine the effects of antioxidants on macular degeneration. The NEI's Age-Related Eye Disease Study (AREDS) is due to be completed by 2005, and involves researchers at eleven clinical centers.

Other promising therapies. Still a long way from general use, these treatments target various characteristics of MD. Matrix metalloproteases (MMPs) are enzymes important in breaking down and remodeling collagen; they may be important in the development of wet MD. The use of oral MMP inhibitors is being investigated for the prevention of wet macular degeneration. Aptamers are molecules designed to target a specific part of the body. An aptamer directed at the cells lining the blood vessels inhibits growth of new blood vessels in animal tumors. Studies are to begin to investigate its potential for the treatment of wet MD. Gene therapy, which replaces the disease-causing genetic mutations with healthy genes, is being investigated for the treatment of both wet and dry MD.

3

Understanding the MD Risk Factors

Many people believe that if a disease or condition "runs in the family," there is nothing they can do to prevent getting it themselves. This is fatalistic and far from the truth. For example, if colon cancer runs in a family, then all members of that family need to get early and regular colonoscopies, change their diet to include more fiber, and reduce the stress in their lives. If colon polyps are detected and removed before they become cancerous, then there is no reason to die. Lifestyle is a significant contributing factor in heart disease, diabetes, and hypertension, and such conditions frequently lead to death when they go hand in hand with high-fat diets, lack of exercise, obesity, and stress. The same is true of macular degeneration.

Cindy, a working mom in her early forties, believed she had always taken care of her health. She enjoyed outdoor activities, especially swimming. On questioning, she acknowledged that she had gotten some bad sunburns in her lifetime and had had sun poisoning on a few occasions. Typically, she did not wear sunglasses. She also admitted to smoking, and to eating lots of meat.

Cindy worked in real estate and spent much of her day listing properties on the local computer network, and laying out advertisements for newspapers. She began to notice that she needed to look more closely at the print on her computer screen, and at the newspaper layouts. At first she compensated by wearing reading glasses that magnified the type she was reading, and by using a brighter light at her desk. However, it became more and more difficult to read even normal-sized print. On her way to and from work, Cindy noticed it was hard to see the road signs because they became distorted and wavy.

When Cindy came to see me, she had a fairly advanced case of macular degeneration, unusual for such a young person. I put her on my MD Four-Step Program of antioxidant supplements, and urged her to change her diet to cut down on the fatty meats and add lots of fresh vegetables. She agreed to stop smoking and wear protective sunglasses, but she was not very optimistic about her chances of regaining her vision.

Cindy let herself be influenced by friends who had a fatalistic attitude and told her that her vision could only get worse, no matter what she did. She resigned from her job, stopped driving, and began to plan for a long-postponed trip to her native Switzerland because she believed it would soon be too late to see any of its beautiful scenery. Depressed as she was, however, Cindy did adhere to my program, and much to her surprise, when she returned from Switzerland she was able to resume driving and reading; best of all, she was able to return to work. Within a year on my program, she was back to 80 percent of her former routine and hoping for a full recovery.

Controlling Your Risk Factors

Your degree of risk is relative to the number of risk factors to which you are exposed. You are in control of most of these. For example, you may be a fair-skinned woman over sixty, which puts you into two risk categories for macular degeneration: age and being female. If you smoke, don't get enough antioxidants, and do not exercise, then you have almost all the risk factors, which means your chance of getting MD is greatly increased. If you are that same woman and you change your diet, quit smoking, protect yourself from sunlight, and join a health club, you have eliminated most of the risk factors. Even if there are many people in your family with MD, you can reduce your risk of developing the disease if you begin early enough to get rid of the risk factors you can control and change your lifestyle.

Although you cannot see it happening, your eye is aging like the rest of your body. When your skin becomes damaged, you can immediately see sunburn or wrinkling and loss of elasticity. Many of the factors that cause aging of your skin can also lead to early aging of your eye, and the development of macular degeneration. The most important factors are oxidative stress, hardening of the arteries, smoking, and exposure to sunlight.

The condition is rarely found in people younger than fifty years of age, but by age sixty-five, approximately 15 percent of the population has macular degeneration. By the age of seventy-five, the number has increased to nearly one in three.

Oxidative stress damages the retinal photoreceptors and the retinal pigment epithelium (RPE). Eventually this damage results in the formation of drusen, retinal pigment epithelial and photoreceptor death, damage to Bruch's membrane, and visual loss. Conditions in the retina are optimal for this type of damage for two reasons. First, the oxygen flow in the retina is higher than at any other site in the body. Second, the retinal photoreceptors contain high concentrations of polyunsaturated fat, which is particularly prone to oxidative damage from free radicals.

By far some of the most potent risk factors for macular degeneration are the ones you totally control: the supplemental nutrients you take, what you eat, whether or not you smoke and exercise, and how well you protect your eyes. When many of my patients were growing up, it was a sign of success to have steak for dinner. Walking went out of fashion when the automobile became king, and women, especially, were never encouraged to be physically active and participate in sports. And, of course, it was cool to smoke cigarettes.

This is beginning to change, but there is still a long way to go. We are gradually becoming more aware, and doctors are including lifestyle changes in their prescriptions, but it can bc difficult to change habits of a lifetime. Look at the risk factors to see which ones are yours.

Lack of Antioxidants

Antioxidants, found in fresh fruit and vegetables, counteract the oxidative wear and tear on your body, and are especially important to your macula. So many studies have demonstrated the effects of a lack of antioxidants that this is no longer controversial or even debatable. Because the macula contains a protective pigment made up of antioxidants, we need to continue to replenish those substances from food and supplements as we age, to offset the breakdown.

Tobacco Smoking

Smoking is responsible for more death and disability than any other single cause, according to the World Health Organization and the Harvard School of Public Health. We all know that smoking causes lung cancer, heart disease, and a wide variety of other ailments, but few people realize that it is absolutely implicated in the development of macular degeneration. Smoking, especially heavy smoking, *increases your risk of macular degeneration two to six times.* Remember, smoking interferes with oxygen transport and utilization; if you smoke, you are depriving your retina of oxygen—not to mention the rest of your body. Smoking constricts the blood vessels, making it more difficult for them to carry nutrients to the organs that need them, including your eyes.

Heavy Alcohol Consumption

Heavy use of alcohol, especially chronic alcoholism, sabotages many of your body's functions. It depletes your supply of zinc and other important antioxidants. It also causes optic neuropathy, a condition of the optic nerve caused by malnutrition. Alcohol interferes with the liver's metabolism and thus with the production of vitamin A, which is essential to the eye.

High-Fat Diet

Arteriosclerosis—the thickening and hardening of the arterial blood vessel wall—is the leading cause of death in the United States and in most westernized societies. The most important cause of arteriosclerosis is the accumulation of fat deposits in the walls of arteries. This is called atherosclerosis.

A study of senior citizens in the Netherlands revealed that people with fat deposits in their arteries were more likely to have age-related macular degeneration than those with clean arteries. Other studies have found that many of the same factors that lead to atherosclerosis also contribute to the development of macular degeneration, including smoking, high blood pressure, and elevated cholesterol levels. Hardening of the arteries reduces the flow of blood and nutrients through the portion of the choroidal blood vessels that supply the retinal pigment epithelium. The RPE becomes damaged and eventually, cells are lost, photoreceptors die, and vision is lost.

Lack of Exercise

More people now understand the health benefits of exercise, and also see that they feel much better when they work out or do some form of physical activity every day. While I am unable to persuade some of my more stubborn patients to join a health club or take up softball or swimming, I have been able to get many to go for a walk at least once every day. Walking is simple, it can be done almost anywhere, and it is one of the most effective aerobic activities.

The delivery of important nutrients to the eye is more limited in a body that does not move. When you walk or move around in other ways, oxygen and blood circulate steadily through your body and keep organs in good condition.

Unprotected Exposure to Sunlight

Sunlight is so powerful that even reflected rays can damage your unprotected eye, particularly light reflected from asphalt, water, or snow. The sun's shortest rays, the ones with the most energy, are called ultraviolet rays. You cannot see them, you cannot feel them, but these are the rays responsible for your suntan. The longest rays, which have the least energy, are the infrared rays that warm you and the environment around you. But it is the rays in the middle, the visible rays responsible for your view of the scenery and the wonderful sunsets, that are responsible for macular degeneration.

The eye focuses all light rays on the retina, but the cornea and lens screen out most of the ultraviolet and infrared. This leaves the visible rays to do most of the damage to the center of the retina—the macula.

High Blood Pressure

Hypertension, often related to hardening of the arteries, affects the blood flow throughout your body—including your eyes—and increases your risk of macular degeneration. Controlling it through diet, exercise, and medications is important and will reduce your risk of heart disease and stroke as well.

Risk Factors You Cannot Control

Heredity

We don't yet know how large a part genetics plays in the development of MD because there are so many potent risk factors, such as your environment, lifestyle, and diet. We do know that siblings, especially twins, of people with macular degeneration are at a higher risk than the general population of developing the condition.

One study has mapped the location of a gene called ARMD1 in one family, but it is too early to tell what this will mean, as far as treatment goes. In order to figure out a genetic linkage analysis you need to look at ten related individuals who have been diagnosed with AMD. What makes this a difficult task is that by the time someone is definitively diagnosed with AMD, they have usually reached the age of sixty or more, their parents are often deceased, and their children are too young to have developed macular degeneration.

In the meantime, even if you come from a family with MD, you are much less likely to develop the disease if you follow my MD Four-Step Program. If you come from a family with several people who have macular degeneration, you should begin getting annual retinal examinations when you are forty years old, and the entire family should be on my MD Four-Step Program.

Race and Iris Color

Most of the studies on macular degeneration have been done in industrialized areas and with mostly white populations. The low proportion of African Americans in such studies has given us the impression that the disease is less prevalent among that group. In the Baltimore Eye Survey, all AMD-related blindness was found in whites, while the leading causes of blindness in blacks were cataracts, glaucoma, diabetic retinopathy, and trauma.

A study of West Indian blacks between forty and eighty-four years of age found features of early age-related macular degeneration common, but still at a lower frequency than in the studies of whites. We are still not sure why this is, but it could be because of the difference in the amount of melanin in their macular pigment. People with abundant melanin in their iris and choroid, such as African Americans, West Indian blacks, and brown-eyed individuals, are less likely to develop visual impairment from age-related macular degeneration than those with fair skin and blue eyes. Apparently the melanin protects against damage from sunlight in the same way it protects the skin, by absorbing radiant energy and displacing it.

A four-year study in Australia revealed that people with blue eyes were twice as likely as those with brown eyes to develop macular degeneration.

Gender

Women develop macular degeneration more frequently than men, although the reason is not completely clear. In one study the incidence of MD in women over seventy-five is 2.2 times greater than in men the same age. A survey of all the existing studies from around the world found a smaller difference, only 1.15 times more women than men, and a study in Denmark found no difference in men and women developing MD. Nevertheless, it does appear more frequently in women.

An old theory has it that men, traditionally the breadwinners, spent more time working indoors and thus had less direct exposure to sunlight. This conclusion is not based on controlled studies, however, and the evidence is only anecdotal. Because clinical studies in the past focused primarily on men, there was a shortage of real knowledge about women's health. This is being remedied since the National Institutes of Health, in the early 1990s, agreed to fund research on women's health equally, and to use women in controlled clinical studies.

We have some evidence that estrogen has been a protective factor for macular degeneration in women, as it has been for heart disease and osteoporosis. Once estrogen production diminishes at menopause, this protective factor diminishes, too. The Eye Disease Case-Control Study found a protective effect from the use of postmenopausal estrogen replacement. The thinking here is that the use of estrogen reduces the risk of heart disease and thus the risk of clogged arteries in the eyes. It may be wise to talk with your internist about taking hormone replacement therapy to lower your risk of macular degeneration—as long as you lower the other risk factors as well, such as bad diet, cigarette smoking, and failure to protect your eyes properly from the sun.

4

Vision and Nutrition: What You Eat Is How You See

Chefs have always believed we eat with our eyes first, and they take pains to present food beautifully. But who thinks the other way around? Do we think of what is good for our eyes when we eat? Except for the old maxim about carrots being good for our eyes (which, by the way, is true), we rarely plan our meals with our eyesight in mind. In this chapter we'll look at how our eyes are affected by nutrition, and specific ways to use this new knowledge will be presented in Part Two.

A link between nutrition and visual function can be traced to 1500 B.C., when improving night vision with nutritional supplements was practiced in Egypt. The active ingredient in those supplements, vitamin A, was discovered in the twentieth century by a Danish physician, C. F. Block. Today there is little question about the importance of vitamin A or its precursor, beta-carotene, to visual function. But vitamin A is not the only nutrient we need for our eyes. Numerous studies from around the world are showing us the protective effect of what we now call antioxidant nutrients on the development of cataracts, macular degeneration, and vascular diseases that can affect the eye.

As mentioned previously, your retina uses more oxygen

than any other part of your body, and the metabolism of this oxygen is vulnerable to disruption because of all the light that filters into your retina. The outer retina is rich in polyunsaturated fatty acids, and can be altered by free radicals and oxidative stress. Therefore you need the protection of nutrients that block that damage. Consider the following:

- In your macula there is a high concentration of lutein and zeaxanthin, two highly protective antioxidants found in green vegetables like spinach and collard greens.
- There is more vitamin E and vitamin C in your eyes than anywhere else in your body.
- There is more of the trace mineral zinc in your retina than anywhere else in your body, and few of us get this in good supply.
- A wall of fat can form under your retina while your arteries are getting clogged, and this prevents the other nutrients from getting through to where they are needed.

The Retina's Need for Antioxidants

If you drive your car for years without any maintenance, the oil becomes sludge and clogs up the engine. This is a result of oxidative stress. A similar thing happens with your body. The fuel keeps getting burned up, but the sludge begins to pile up. The sad fact is that most people take better care of their cars than their bodies. The macula is battered by free radicals, and drusen—a kind of sludge—builds up. Because the retina uses more oxygen than any other part of our body, this oxidative stress is extreme. However, when you get enough antioxidants from supplements and your diet, they prevent the free radicals from wreaking havoc. Free radicals are highly reactive molecules or atoms that attack other molecules, multiplying in the process, and damage tissues. An excess of free radicals is one of the leading causes of cataracts and macular degeneration, as well as of the aging process in general.

Antioxidants are naturally occurring substances (mainly vitamins C and E, beta-carotene, lutein, and zeaxanthin) that help destroy free radicals that lead to oxidative stress and potential loss of vision. They are like the body's environmental police.

Despite our growing knowledge of the importance of antioxidant vitamins and minerals on visual function, and on the body as a whole, the medical community has maintained for years that if you eat a balanced diet, nutritional supplements and special diets are not necessary. This is not true.

As long ago as 1958, we saw the first evidence of the beneficial effect of vitamins in treating macular degeneration. Study subjects received either a placebo (nonmedicated substance) or vitamin E. Researchers thought a reduction in distortion, and an improvement of two lines of vision, could be considered a positive response. An amazing two-thirds of the subjects who received the vitamin supplements showed this positive response! However, *it was another thirty years* before more research was performed.

- In 1988 the first National Health and Nutrition Examination Survey of people over forty-five years of age found that those who ate a diet rich in beta-carotene were less likely to develop MD than those who did not.
- In 1993 researchers at Harvard University and Johns Hopkins University found that Americans with lower blood levels of the antioxidants beta-carotene, vitamins C and E, and selenium, or those with high serum cholesterol levels, *had a higher incidence of macular degeneration.* In 1994, the same researchers found eating a diet rich in carotenoids, as compared with one low in carotenoids, reduced the risk of MD by 43 percent. Among the carotenoids, lutein and zeaxanthin, found

in high concentrations in spinach and collard greens, were most strongly associated with a decreased risk. Those people who ate spinach or collard greens five to six times a week or more, compared with those who ate these less than once a month, were 88 percent less likely to develop MD.

- The Baltimore Longitudinal Study of Aging found that high levels of vitamin E offered a protective effect against MD, as did an "antioxidant index" of vitamin C, vitamin E, and beta-carotene combined.
- As part of the 1995 Beaver Dam (Wisconsin) Eye Study, researchers found that very low levels of lycopene (the most abundant antioxidant found in the body) were associated with a higher risk of MD.
- In 1996 a Chicago study found that antioxidant vitamin supplements reduced the progression of MD over a period of one and a half years.

Although the studies do not agree on the most effective level of antioxidants in the blood, there is clearly evidence that low blood levels are associated with a higher degree of MD. Equally important to note is that no study found people with higher levels to be at higher risk for macular degeneration.

These and other studies, taken together, provide compelling evidence of the association between nutrition and vision. Your risk of developing macular degeneration can actually be reduced by as much as 80 percent in some cases! And, to derive the maximum benefit from the research, it is important to begin with your daily diet, since supplements alone may or may not deliver the key components of the foods they represent. A number of studies have compared the incidence and severity of macular degeneration and cataracts with intake of vitamin supplements, and have found that people taking supplements had a lower risk of MD, and that the disease was less severe.

We need antioxidants in our diet, but some need to be taken in supplement form because we cannot get enough in our diet. Let's take a closer look at the particular antioxidants we need: lutein and zeaxanthin, beta-carotene, and vitamins C and E.

But first let's define carotenoids and beta-carotene.

- A carotenoid is any of several plant and animal pigments related to and including beta-carotene. Lutein and zeaxanthin are also carotenoids, but they are more often found in green vegetables rather than red or yellow ones. Lutein and zeaxanthin must be obtained from our diet.
- Beta-carotene, also a carotenoid, is any of several red- or orange-colored organic compounds found in carrots and other vegetables. It is changed into vitamin A in the liver during the digestive process.

In 1945 the yellow pigment in the macula was identified as a carotenoid, but it wasn't until much later that we discovered that these carotenoids are also present in some green leafy vegetables. These yellow pigments, lutein and zeaxanthin, can filter out blue light and protect the retina from photic damage. The multicenter Eye Disease Case-Control Study sponsored by the National Eye Institute discovered and reported this in the *Journal of the American Medical Association* in 1994.

Lutein and Zeaxanthin, "Nature's Sunglasses"

I call the carotenoids lutein and zeaxanthin "nature's sunglasses," and with good reason. These two antioxidant compounds, which are found abundantly in leafy green vegetables such as spinach and kale, form the xanthophyll pigment in the human macula, which absorbs the specific visible light rays that damage the macula. This pigment gives the region its name—macula lutea. Among the fourteen dietary carotenoids routinely detected in human blood, only lutein and zeaxanthin accumulate in the retina at much higher concentrations than other equally prominent carotenoids such as lycopene, alpha-carotene, and beta-carotene.

A number of companies are now marketing artificial supplements with the promise that they will be equally effective. But until we know for sure that artificial carotenoid supplements will do the same job as diet, we should stick with what we know works for this nutrient—your diet. We need supplements for zinc and vitamins C and E, but not for lutein and zeaxanthin.

Although maximizing your intake of other antioxidants, such as vitamins C and E and zinc, is important, they are a less important focus of your meal plan and diet, since your intake of these will be boosted safely with supplements (see chapter 6).

Lutein and zeaxanthin are also powerful antioxidants that reduce oxidative stress in the most highly metabolic of areas—your macula. Interestingly, lutein and zeaxanthin are not nearly so important or apparent in the peripheral macula. Lutein and zeaxanthin are also in your eye's lens, and may protect you against cataracts as well. Although lutein is an abundant carotenoid in green and some yellow fruits and vegetables, the dietary sources of zeaxanthin are limited to corn, peaches, some squash varieties, and citrus fruit. Romaine lettuce is the only green leafy vegetable with moderate concentrations of zeaxanthin. Also, your body cannot make its own lutein, but it can make zeaxanthin from lutein, so what you eat plays a very big role in having enough of these antioxidants.

I recommend getting lutein and zeaxanthin from your diet, because there is no solid evidence that supplements work, and only one of them is commercially available. Currently lutein is isolated and purified commercially from extracts of marigold flowers. We still have no way of isolating and producing zeaxanthin.

Beta-carotene

While lutein is found almost entirely in green vegetables, beta-carotene is found in both green and yellow and orange vegetables and fruit. The best source of beta-carotene is the lowly carrot! As children, many of us were told that carrots help us see in the dark, and now we have scientific proof that carrots do help to preserve vision.

It is particularly important to maximize your dietary intake of this group of antioxidants, because high doses of supplemental beta-carotene have been found to cause more harm than good in some cases. On the other hand, natural beta-carotene obtained from food has been found to be highly beneficial in preserving vision, and preventing other medical problems such as cancer. It is likely that the reason for this is that there are other nutrients in the foods rich in beta-carotene that have not yet been identified but that are responsible for their beneficial effect.

Foods with a high beta-carotene content, in addition to carrots, include sweet potatoes, dried or raw apricots, beet greens, cantaloupe, mango, mustard greens, dried peaches, pumpkin, and winter squash. There is beta-carotene in meat, but this is not a good source because, in meat, it is converted into vitamin A. The goal is to get beta-carotene before it becomes vitamin A.

Vitamins C and E: The Eyes Have Most of It

Your eyes need a great deal of these two potent antioxidants, vitamin C and vitamin E, because they are a natural part of the structure of your eye.

Vitamin C: Not Just for Colds

The ascorbic acid (vitamin C) level in the eye's aqueous humor and lens may exceed the level in your blood by more than fifty times. We know that people with cataracts have less ascorbic acid in their eyes than do those with normal eyes. Ascorbic acid is a white crystalline substance, similar in structure to glucose, and is easily destroyed by oxidation and heat.

Since the Nobel Prize–winning chemist Linus Pauling published his findings about vitamin C in the late 1960s, it has been a controversial vitamin as a supplement. Many of us know that vitamin C prevents scurvy and protects us against colds, but few of us realize how important it is for our eyes. Vitamin C works together with vitamin E to protect our retinal pigment epithelium (RPE) from the damage of free radicals, and thus oxidation. It is suspected that vitamin C deprivation may be a factor in diabetic retinal hemorrhages, and the formation of cataracts, too.

Many of us believe our morning glass of orange juice takes care of our vitamin C requirements. I saw a funny television commercial from an orange juice producer. At breakfast, a man sits before a tiny glass—hardly bigger than a whiskey shot glass—and complains that this is not enough orange juice. Next, he is chugalugging the juice directly from the container. However, even if you drink the entire half-gallon container, it will not be enough to protect you from the ravages of oxidation. In order to get the vitamin C you need every day, you would have to drink twelve eight-ounce glasses of orange juice. Or you could eat ten cups of frozen strawberries or ten cups of boiled broccoli. This would be difficult, to say the least, and possibly unwise, even for those of us in the best of health.

One way to increase your dietary vitamin C is to take a supplement with your orange juice. To preserve your vision you will need to take 1,000 mg of vitamin C daily. This may be hard to do with diet alone, as we have seen, unless you drink one-half cup of acerola juice. Known as the Barbados cherry, acerola is extraordinarily high in natural vitamin C; however, it is not easy to find the product, even in health-food stores. (Chewable acerola tablets are available in some stores.)

Unlike vitamins A and E, vitamin C is water-soluble. This means that it is much harder to overdose on vitamin C supplements because the excess just gets flushed out. Too much, however, can produce side effects such as diarrhea and heartburn.

Foods we eat regularly that are high in vitamin C include cantaloupe, cranberry juice, grapefruit juice, lemon juice, oranges, guavas, papayas, red peppers, and strawberries. Orange juice also makes a great fresh salad dressing ingredient and, for a light orange flavor, can be used in place of half the water when cooking rice. You can add nutrients and vitamin C to salads by topping them with fresh strawberries or chopped papaya, kiwi, or red pepper.

Vitamin E: The Fountain of Youth

Natural vitamin E concentrations increase in your RPE and peripheral retina and macula until you are around fifty years old. Then it levels off and begins to decrease after the age of seventy. The rod outer segments and the RPE layers in the retina have the highest concentrations of vitamin E. These tissues are usually the last to give up their concentrations of vitamin E during dietary deprivation, and are particularly sensitive to oxidation.

Oxidation is very dynamic within the retina because the oxygen flow to the RPE photoreceptor complex is higher than at any other site in the body. Vitamin E is the major, if not the only, chain-breaking antioxidant, and is a major scavenger of free radicals.

Vitamin E may indeed be the magic bullet of vitamins. One of the most potent of antioxidants for fighting off disease, it exists in many forms, but alpha-tocopherol is the most commonly synthesized form. This is a viscous oil that is not water-soluble. It is stable in heat, but is readily destroyed by oxidation and ultraviolet light. Research shows that high levels of alpha-tocopherol in the blood are protective against age-related MD.

Zinc: The Retina's Power Mineral

How often do you eat a half-dozen oysters on the half shell? If you did, you would probably get enough zinc from your diet. However, you are not likely to do this unless you live on the Chesapeake Bay, so you will probably do well to take a zinc supplement.

I find it ironic that the two functions that most require adequate zinc are sight and sex. Oysters, for example, have been considered an aphrodisiac for hundreds of years, but it has only recently been found that the prostate gland needs lots of zinc to manufacture semen. Our eyes need zinc even more. This mineral is found in highest concentrations in our eyes (and then in the prostate and semen). When we don't ingest enough zinc, then our eyes have less to work with.

Zinc is the second most abundant trace element in the body, but the most abundant in the eye, especially in the retina, where it plays a key role in metabolism and is essential for oxidation. Zinc also makes it possible for vitamin A to be released from the liver in order to form rhodopsin in the retina. Lack of zinc can prevent the photoreceptors from functioning. Zinc is necessary for the activity of more than one hundred enzymes, and is essential for cell membrane stability and immune function.

Classic signs of insufficient zinc include not only night blindness but also growth retardation, delayed sexual maturity, anorexia, depressed taste acuity, impaired immune function, and slow wound healing.

The body's zinc supply can be depleted by many things, including the phosphates in carbonated drinks, diuretics, laxatives, iron supplements, and by too much cereal protein. Zinc levels can also be depressed by taking steroids and oral contraceptives. Zinc can also become depleted owing to alcoholism and other conditions such as diabetes or renal failure.

Unlike the other antioxidants, higher concentrations of zinc are found in meat and seafood than in vegetables and fruit. Zinc is absorbed more easily from red meat, poultry, and fish than from fruits and vegetables. It is estimated that 43 percent of zinc in the U.S. food supply is from meat, fish, and poultry, and 25 percent from dairy products. Good sources include beef, lamb, liver, oysters, and veal.

Although some vegetables have moderate amounts of zinc, legumes such as lentils and lima beans, and grains such as oatmeal and wheat germ are the best sources. If you are a vegetarian, then understand that fruits and vegetables provide less than 0.5 mg of zinc per serving. That's why zinc supplements are an important part of my MD Four-Step Program.

Zinc interacts extensively with other minerals, particularly copper. This begins in the digestive tract, where the two bind together. Too much zinc can wipe out the necessary trace mineral copper, so both are taken together to avoid this loss. Zinc is excreted through the digestive system.

As with vitamin E and vitamin C, getting enough zinc from your diet alone is difficult unless you eat four raw oysters (from an *unpolluted* bay) every day, which is not recommended due to the risk of getting hepatitis A or a potentially deadly bacterial infection. Otherwise, you would need to eat roughly one and a half pounds of the next best source, calf's liver, every day, or a one-and-a-half-pound sirloin steak, and that would be a heart attack on a plate.

The current RDA for zinc is 15 mg, but this assumes that 40 percent of what you get in your diet is absorbed. I recommend getting 45 mg of zinc from supplements, and then up to 55 mg more from your diet. Though zinc is important for our body's own antioxidant and visual systems, care must be exercised, since high levels of zinc may increase the risk of Alzheimer's disease.

Trace Minerals

Copper, selenium, and manganese are other nutrients essential to the eye.

Copper

Copper is necessary because of its activity with enzymes, and because it works with vitamin C to combat oxidative stress. The liver, kidney, heart, and brain contain the highest concentrations of copper. It is important to take this if you are taking zinc supplements, because zinc can create a deficiency of copper, which can lead to anemia, growth retardation, defective keratinization and pigmentation of hair, hypothermia, degenerative changes in the larger blood vessels, mental deterioration, and skeletal changes. Alternatively, excessive copper intake can lead to hepatitis, cirrhosis, tremor, mental deterioration, deposits in your cornea, hemolytic anemia, and renal dysfunction, so you do not want to overdo it. USRDA ranges are from 0.4 mg a day for babies to 2.0 mg a day for adults. Food sources of copper include seafood, mushrooms, beans, lentils, some nuts, and wheat germ.

Selenium

Selenium is an important cofactor for an enzyme crucial in preventing oxidative stress, particularly the breakdown of hydrogen peroxide. A deficiency of this mineral is known to lead to cataracts. It also cures or prevents a condition characterized by heart disease and nerve damage; this was discovered because that condition is endemic in a province of China where the soil is deficient in this mineral. Selenium toxicity causes hair loss, abnormal nails, emotional lability, lassitude, and a "garlic" breath. Necessary for preventing oxidative stress, selenium works with vitamin E in regulating the free radicals. Selenium is found in fish and seafood, whole grains, legumes, wheat germ, mushrooms, and tofu.

Manganese

Manganese is an activator for important antioxidant enzymes. Deficiency is rare in humans, but has caused abnormalities of the skeletal systems, central nervous systems, and reproductive systems of animals. There is one report of a human bleeding disorder traced to a manganese deficiency. Too much manganese over long periods of time can result in anorexia, apathy, headaches, impotence, leg cramps, and speech disturbances. It is found in whole grains such as oats, and in nuts, seeds, seaweed, and some vegetables. Manganese has been leaching out of the soil in the United States, most severely in the Southeast.

Blocked Arteries: The Heart and Eye Connection

The retina is a lipid-rich environment, which means there are lots of fatty acids present in it; when these are exposed to light and oxygen, the potential for oxidative stress is great. This is why we need such a high quantity of antioxidants to maintain the integrity of this tissue. Without these antioxidants to balance the dynamics of the oxygen, oxidative stress occurs, and macular degeneration develops.

Many people who have heart disease—atherosclorosis, or clogged arteries—also have macular degeneration. There are two likely reasons for this. The first is that a high-fat diet that causes the arteries to the heart to get clogged can do the same for the arteries to the eyes. This reduces the nutrient-rich (antioxidant-rich) blood flow. The other possible reason is that excess fat may deposit itself in the tissues behind the retina. If the latter is the case, then nutrients cannot pass through the "wall of fat" to reach the cells that nourish the retina.

Atherosclerosis, as we know, is associated with dietary intake of cholesterol and saturated fat, cigarette smoking, hypertension, obesity, diabetes, and physical inactivity. Again, the researchers found that those with advanced atherosclerosis were at least two to four times more likely than those without it to have macular degeneration. The National Health and Nutrition Examination Survey found that people with a history of vascular disease, particularly those who had suffered a stroke, were also more likely to have macular degeneration.

Early research suggests that if your diet includes too much saturated fat (basically animal fat, such as butter, lard, fatty meat, and full-fat dairy products), then you have an 80 percent greater chance of developing early AMD than do those who do not have a high-fat diet. As you learned earlier, the area around the macula begins to break down. Not everyone who develops the early stage will develop the late stage, but your chance is much greater. Why risk it?

In chapter 14 you will find ways to trim the fat in your diet, and chapter 15 contains some exercise programs.

5

The Light in Your Eyes

The eyes are the windows of the soul. They are also the windows through which too much light pours, unless you pull down the shades once in a while. It is because of all this light coming through that your eyes are exposed to high levels of oxidative stress that can bring on macular degeneration.

There was a time when I, along with most mainstream doctors, believed that sunlight caused little damage to vision, even without sunglasses. The eye, we believed, was protected by the pupil, which constricts in response to bright light, reducing the amount of light entering the eye. The pupil dilates in darker conditions and lets in more light. In fact, we had concerns about recommending sunglasses because, we thought, by blocking light, the dark lens would make the pupil dilate. Then, if the sunglasses did a poor job of screening out harmful rays, they would actually do more harm than good.

When I moved to the Sunshine State, I was intrigued by the high incidence of both cataracts and macular degeneration in people who had spent most of their lives outdoors in almost constant sunshine. It seemed that sunlight was a factor, but which element of sunlight was the true culprit?

The sun emits a broad spectrum of energy (electromagnetic radiation), some of which we can see, some of which we can feel, and some of which we can neither see nor feel. The most powerful (and potentially the most damaging) rays are the ones with the shortest wavelengths and the greatest energy. Fortunately, the earth's atmosphere filters out most of these—although the ozone layer is not protecting us as well as it used to.

The energy, and thus the potential for damage to our eyes, is inversely proportional to solar wavelengths. This means that the shorter wavelengths, like ultraviolet, have more energy than the longer wavelengths, like infrared. Extremely short wavelengths, which include X rays and cosmic rays, are highly dangerous, while the longer radio waves are harmless (see figure 5.1).

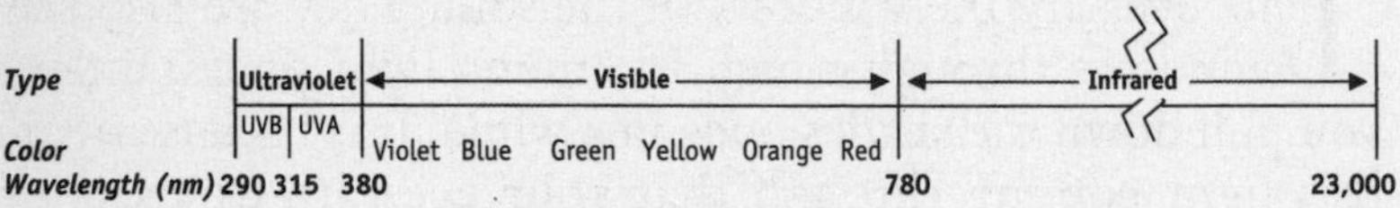

Figure 5.1. Sunlight.

Most of the solar radiation reaching the surface of the earth is infrared, the longest wavelengths that we can feel as heat, but that we don't see. About one-third of the radiation is in the middle wavelength, or the visible spectrum, which allows us to see and makes the sky appear blue. Only 5 percent of all light striking the globe is in the ultraviolet (UV) range, the shortest wavelengths. In short, then, ultraviolet burns, infrared heats, and visible light lets us see.

Ultraviolet, Infrared, and Visible Light

Ultraviolet Light (UV)

Ultraviolet light (UV) is divided into three subgroups, of which UVA is the mildest and most abundant, constituting 97 percent of all UV radiation, and UVC the strongest. Only UVA and UVB light reach the earth through the atmosphere, because UVC is filtered out. It is ultraviolet rays that cause skin to burn. Ultraviolet radiation is strongest at high altitudes, near the equator, and in open or reflective environments, such as snow, water, or sand (more about this later). UV light is primarily absorbed by the front surface of your eye, the cornea and lens. This can result in eye irritation and the early formation of cataracts, but it does not result in a permanent reduction in vision unless the cataracts are left untreated. A small amount of UV light does reach the retina after most is filtered by the cornea and lens. This occurs mostly in children and seniors who have undergone cataract surgery and did not receive a lens implant that blocks UV light.

In children, up to 8 percent of some UV light is transmitted to the retina. By the age of twenty-two, this diminishes to less than one-tenth of 1 percent. Because the retina is six times more sensitive to damage from UV light than any other kind, even this small amount of UV light needs to be taken seriously and blocked before it gets into your eyes.

Infrared Light (IR)

Infrared light is thermal radiation, i.e., heat. While you are sitting in the sun, your arm may feel hot from this light, but it is getting burned by the UV light. Infrared light has not been found to be an important factor in the development of macular degeneration, but it has been implicated in the formation of cataracts. IR is partly absorbed by clouds, moisture, dust, carbon dioxide, and other gases in the atmosphere, reducing its levels before it reaches the earth. But while you might feel less heat on a cloudy day, the ultraviolet rays are still getting through, and your eyes need protection.

Visible Light

Visible light is that part of the sun's energy we experience as daylight. It is a spectrum of different colors of light, each color with a corresponding wavelength. Visible light is one of the leading causes of macular degeneration because so much of it reaches the retina.

Your eyelids protect you to some extent, in that they automatically shut if you stare directly into the sun. Your eye is affected by the degree to which your eyes are open. When you squint, your upper and lower lids block 95 percent of light reaching your eyes. When you look at the ground, however, your lids are usually opened wider, and this way you are vulnerable to reflected light.

The amount of solar radiation that reaches us on the earth's surface varies according to location, altitude, sky cover, time of day, and time of the year. If we compare Atlanta and El Paso, which are at the same latitude, we find that El Paso gets about 38 percent more solar radiation because it is in a higher and dryer region of the country. If we compare Hawaii and Alaska, we find that Hawaii receives about ten times more solar radiation than Alaska because it's closer to the equator.

Time of Day

Time of day has a great deal to do with the amount of solar exposure your eyes get. The greatest amount of UV exposure occurs when the sun is directly overhead at noon. Its force is ten times greater at that time than three hours before or after the local solar noon. In summer, a person with fair skin would receive a mild sunburn in twenty-five minutes at noon, but would have to lie in the sun for at least two hours to get the same burn three hours later.

If you are in the sun all day—from 8:00 A.M. to 4:00 P.M.—you will receive 40 percent of the total UV exposure for only two hours, from 11:00 A.M. to 1:00 P.M. From 10:00 A.M. to 2:00 P.M. you get a whopping 72 percent. So it might be a good idea to think of something to do indoors during this period of the day.

When the sun is overhead and white, it would take only 90 seconds of staring at the sun to receive a solar retinitis, or "eclipse burn." A few hours later, with the sun much lower in the sky, it would take several minutes to reach a hazardous retinal dose, and it is virtually impossible at sunset.

Reflected Light

Most of the damaging light is reflected light, because we never actually look directly into the sun. When I play golf I rarely wear sunglasses, just a hat with a brim. Although I am looking at the ground a lot, there is little reflected light on a green golf course. However, a parking lot attendant, working on asphalt all day, is bombarded with ten times more reflected light than I am on the golf course. And a skier gets eighty-eight times more reflected light than the golfer. Obviously, there is an enormous amount of light reflected on snow and water.

Light reflected off the ground plays the greatest role in determining how much sunlight is getting into your eyes. The greatest exposure is from ground reflections from snow, which reflects 88 percent of the light, followed by sea foam/surf (27 percent), dry beach sand (17 percent), concrete pavement (10 percent), black asphalt (7 percent), and a wooden boat deck (6 percent). There is little effect from looking at the horizon, the sky, green grass, or foliage.

The angle at which light can enter the eye through our lids when we are squinting on a sunny day is approximately 10 degrees; on a slightly overcast day when we squint less it is 10 to 30 degrees. For the most part, when we are walking we are looking down. As a result, at the middle of the day, when sunlight is at its strongest and the most damaging, it typically cannot directly enter the eye. Reflected light, however, can enter the eye, and becomes significantly more important. In addition, by using a visor or a brimmed hat, which means a hat with a brim of two and a half inches or more, you can eliminate virtually all the direct sunlight. This leaves reflected sunlight as the most important determinant of how important wearing sunglasses will be to you.

Hundreds of cases of MD were observed in young men

in military service in regions of intense sunlight. The condition developed over several months and was most severe when bright sunlight was reflected from water or sand. In another study of thousands of men in Southeast Asia during World War II, the effects of the intense sunlight were made more serious because malnutrition apparently reduced the efficiency of their eyes' defense mechanisms.

Before we had the equipment to measure and document the amount of UV light reflected and directly hitting our eye, we still had to cope with snow blindness. In fact, the Inuit (Eskimo) people long ago knew how to protect themselves from the arctic snow. They invented their own "sunglasses" made of whalebone. These shields were similar in shape to a regular pair of large sunglasses, with big round lenses of opque whalebone. A thin horizontal slit, less than a quarter-inch high, crossed the middle of the lens. The wearer's eyes were completely protected from rays above the line of sight and from those reflected from snow and ice below. The only light that got in was directly in front of their line of vision. When these devices were tested for UV protection when the wearer was looking off into the horizon during the middle of the day, they blocked over 99 percent of UV light. Cloth masks or veils with slits are used in a similar manner by certain nomadic tribes in the desert when out in the midday sun.

The Color of Light

When I turned my attention to studies on sunlight and macular degeneration, I had a surprise: the findings are decidedly different from those for cataracts, which are caused by UV light. Macular degenaration is caused by visible light, particularly the shorter blue wavelengths.

Cataracts, in a sense, are our own natural sunglasses. In addition to UV protection of the retina, they often block the blue wavelengths. Thus, when a cataract is surgically removed, the protection is removed with it. The intraocular lens that is then inserted into the eye does not always have UV protection built in, and never provides protection against blue wavelengths.

In one study, the amount of time that men spent outdoors in summer was linked with a higher risk of both early and late macular degeneration. But here a protective effect was found from wearing a hat or sunglasses—or both—that shield the eyes from visible light. Exposure to UV light did not appear to have any effect. Could this be true? If UV light did not contribute to the development of macular degeneration, were we being led to a false sense of security by simply wearing sunglasses we thought offered 100-percent UV protection? It appeared so.

The importance of visible light, particularly the shorter blue wavelengths, on the development of macular degeneration was discovered by Dr. Hugh R. Taylor, a professor of ophthalmology at Johns Hopkins University. Chesapeake Bay watermen were chosen to study because their work in catching crabs, oysters, and other seafood from the bay meant they were out in open boats year round, exposed to light made more intense by its reflection off water. Most of these men do not wear sunglasses because the lenses get covered with salt spray from the water and block their vision. The only ones who did wear glasses were men who needed to wear prescription glasses. (Ironically, these men were gathering shellfish, which are among the best sources of zinc, which would help protect them from macular degeneration.)

In 1666, Isaac Newton helped us define light by showing us colors that we now know as wavelengths of energy. Each wavelength affects the eye differently (see figure 5.2).

Rainbows and glass prisms separate this white light into colors, beginning with violet, which has the shortest wavelength, through blue, green, yellow, orange, and finally red, which has the longest wavelength. Because of their greater energy, the shortest wavelengths of visible light—violet and

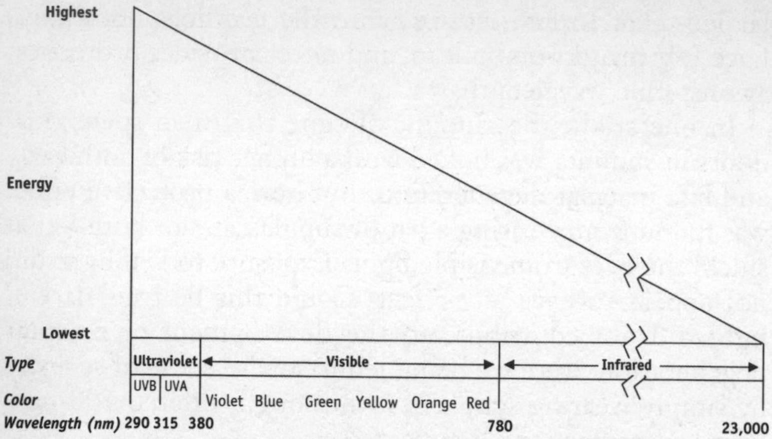

Figure 5.2. The Composition of Sunlight.
Sunlight represents a spectrum of energy. The shorter the wavelength, the higher the energy and the greater the potential damage to your vision.

blue—can do damage to the eye with a much smaller amount of light, as little as one-tenth of that needed by light at a longer wavelength, such as red.

The back of the eye, mainly the macula, is the only part that seems to be susceptible to visible light, particularly the shorter blue wavelengths. The retina contains specific chromophores in the photoreceptor rods, cones, RPE, and choroid, whose job is to absorb visible light. As the intensity of the light increases and its wavelength gets shorter (with ultraviolet and blue light in particular), the eye is less able to absorb the light without damage.

Other Dangers from Light

Ozone: The Earth's Imperfect Sunglasses

The damage to our ozone layer makes us more vulnerable to the dangers of solar radiation because more of it can now come through. Ozone is an extra-thick layer of oxygen wrapped around the earth to protect it from solar radiation. It acts on the globe the way sunglasses act on us. Ozone is a molecule of oxygen comprising three atoms, as opposed to normal oxygen, which contains two atoms. It is created when oxygen in the stratosphere is bombarded by ultraviolet radiation from the sun. Because this layer—or filter—is getting weaker owing to industrial abuse, our exposure to UV light is on the rise. NASA scientists report that from 1978 to 1984 there was a 3-percent reduction in the ozone layer. In recent years, reductions in the layer of 15 to 25 percent have been measured in Ann Arbor, Michigan; New York City; and other parts of the world.

The amount of UV light that reaches the retina is greatest in children and in people who have had cataract surgery, so protection is even more important for these groups. Since UV radiation exposure before ten years of age is known as the leading determinant of skin cancer, it is likely that protecting children's eyes from UV and visible light is of equal importance. We should shield the eyes of the very young with good-quality sunglasses.

Fortunately, there is a simple solution. UV exposure can be reduced by wearing protective lenses that block 100 percent of UV light and a brimmed hat (see chapter 17).

PART II

THE MD FOUR-STEP PROGRAM

GETTING STARTED

The MD Four-Step Program will prevent the degeneration of your macula and thus your vision. The program is easy to follow, and the only expense involved is for nutritional supplements and better sunglasses. It is designed to reduce risk factors and lead you to a lifestyle that will strengthen and protect your general health as well as your vision. The following chapters give you everything you will need to accomplish the program's four steps.

Step 1. Take Five Nutritional Supplements

Take these supplements because some nutrients are difficult to get in your diet. Vitamins C and E, beta-carotene, and the minerals zinc, selenium, and manganese are elements we already consume in small quantities; they simply need to be supplemented.

Step 2. Begin a Diet Rich in Antioxidants and Low in Fat

Eat fruits and green leafy vegetables, which are easy to increase in the diet when they are prepared in nutritious and appetizing recipes.

Step 3. Eliminate Risk Factors with a Healthful Lifestyle

Stop smoking and heavy alcohol consumption and incorporate regular, moderate exercise to help eliminate risk factors.

Step 4. Protect Your Eyes from Visible Light

Learn to choose sunglasses that will give you the protection you need from visible light as well as UV, and will be suitable for various environments and activities.

Before you begin the MD Four-Step Program, check with your doctor to make sure it won't interact negatively with any medication you are taking. And remember, this program will protect you not only from macular degeneration, but from many other disorders as well.

STEP 1

TAKE FIVE NUTRITIONAL SUPPLEMENTS

6

Guidelines for Taking Vitamin and Mineral Supplements

Although many vitamins and minerals can be obtained from your diet, supplements are necessary to reach the intake levels needed to preserve vision. More important, by *not* taking the recommended minimum amounts in supplement form, you are not getting the full benefit of these nutrients for your vision. So unless you experience unwanted side effects, or if your doctor tells you not to take supplements for medical reasons, aim to get these recommended amounts by taking supplements.

The supplement levels recommended in my MD Four-Step Program are well within the known safety range. While there are slight differences in the needs of adult men and women, they are not significant enough to concern us. The only exception would be a woman's higher need for iron and calcium at various times of her life.

An abundance of research supports taking antioxidants at higher levels than the U.S. Recommended Daily Allowance (RDA), if we want to build a strong defense against the free radicals and oxidative stress that can harm our vision. The fact is, we simply cannot absorb enough antioxidants through our daily diet. To get 1,000 mg of vitamin C, we would have to eat twelve to twenty-three oranges or more than two pounds of broccoli. Even if we were to eat eight to ten generous portions of fruits and vegetables each day, which most of us do not, it is simply not possible to get enough vitamin E from our diet. We would have to eat more nuts, almonds, whole grains, hazelnut oil, or other vitamin-E-rich foods than our systems could readily handle. For example, to get 400 IU of vitamin E daily, we would need eight cups of hazelnut oil, eight cups of almonds, or four cups of sunflower seeds. The fat and calorie content would be enormous—for the hazelnut oil alone, it would be over 6,000 calories! So, obviously, the best way to ensure that we get the antioxidants we need is to take supplements.

The chart of Daily Vitamin and Mineral Supplement Recommendations on page 70 was developed from the latest scientific information available on optimal amounts of beta-carotene, vitamin C, vitamin E, zinc, selenium, copper, and manganese needed to preserve your vision and health. My recommendation is to get these amounts from supplements, and then to augment this through dietary intake. The main reason for not taking more in the form of supplements is that the latest studies show no benefit from taking higher doses of supplements, and higher doses may cause problems, as we will see with beta-carotene. Instead, you will further increase your antioxidant intake through your diet, as described in subsequent chapters. Now, before rushing out to buy supplements, here's a review of each nutrient you need in the form of supplements.

Daily Requirements

BETA-CAROTENE 5,000 IU; RDA: 5,000 IU

Beta-carotene is a potent antioxidant that your body converts to vitamin A, which is essential for vision. By taking beta-carotene supplements rather than vitamin A, you get the added power of an antioxidant along with the vitamin A you need for your vision. Beta-carotene is also less toxic than vitamin A.

Take just 5,000 IU of beta-carotene (the U.S. Recommended Daily Allowance for vitamin A, into which beta-carotene is converted) in supplement form and get the rest through your diet. (See subsequent chapters for food sources.)

Cautions. Because of their power, beta-carotene supplements must be taken with care. High doses have been associated with a higher rate of lung cancer in smokers. Beta-carotene can also accumulate under your skin and cause discoloration. High doses may also be toxic when taken in combination with alcohol.

Vitamin C 1,000 mg; RDA: 60mg

Vitamin C is easily destroyed in food while it is being shipped or prepared, so you need to supplement your diet with 1,000 mg daily. Consider breaking this amount into two doses of 500 mg, or four 250-mg doses. This may help you to maximize absorption of the vitamin. Don't take chewable vitamin C because this form produces an acid that can dissolve tooth enamel. Tablets are best. Vitamin C can be made synthetically or come from natural sources, such as rose hips. Although rose hips are relatively high in vitamin C, this dried fruit has widely variable amounts of vitamin C, and labels do not usually show how much is synthetic and how much is natural. Since rose-hip-derived vitamin C is twenty-five times more expensive to extract than synthetic vitamin C is to make, it is easy to understand why most vitamin C is synthetic.

Water-soluble vitamin C flushes out of your system if your intake exceeds what your body needs. That is why megadoses of vitamin C are a waste of money; all you end up with is expensive urine.

Cautions. One study found a possible harmful effect of vitamin C supplementation, an increased risk of one type of cataract. To my knowledge there are no other data that show any harmful effect for vitamin C, so I stick with my recommendation for including vitamin C. And remember, even if this one negative finding is upheld, cataracts can be treated with a simple surgical procedure! Macular degeneration is much more difficult to treat, and remains the leading cause of vision loss in the United States and Western Europe.

Vitamin C in very high doses—4,000 mg or more daily—may cause stomach irritation, loose stools, or diarrhea. (Diarrhea has been known to occur with doses as low as 500 mg a day.) Should any of these happen, even at lower doses, reduce your intake until the problem clears up. Also, because vitamin C is excreted through the kidneys, people with a history of kidney stones should exercise caution when taking doses larger than the RDA of 60 mg a day.

VITAMIN E 400 IU; RDA: 30 IU

It is not likely or even practical to get adequate amounts of vitamin E from your diet, and I recommend a supplement of 400 IU daily, in addition to a dietary intake of up to 100 IU a day. (See subsequent chapters for food sources of this important antioxidant.)

There is some evidence that natural vitamin E is more effective than the synthetic version. It is also more expensive. However, some versions labeled as natural may contain only 20 percent natural and 80 percent synthetic vitamin E. If you decide to buy natural vitamin E, read the labels carefully. Natural vitamin E is *d*-alpha tocopherol. Synthetic vitamin E is *dl*-alpha-tocopherol. You may also see the words "acetate" or "succinate," as in "dl-alpha-tocopherol acetate." These types are believed by some to be more active than other forms.

Cautions. Vitamin E itself acts as a blood thinner, so if your doctor has put you on medication such as Coumadin or aspirin, you should check before taking it. Also consult your doctor if you are taking omega-3 fatty acids (fish oils), as they also act to thin the blood. Vitamin E may also cause a rise in your cholesterol level, so it's a good idea to have your cholesterol level checked at least annually.

Take only recommended levels of vitamin E, which is fat-soluble but, unlike vitamin A, has not been shown to build up to toxic levels. Nevertheless, we don't recommend high levels because excess amounts may interfere with the absorption and function of other fat-soluble vitamins. While 400 IU of vitamin E is well above the RDA of 30 IU, it is considered safe.

Zinc 45mg; RDA: 15mg

As you now know, zinc is the second-most-common trace element in the body, and the most abundant element in the eye. It is essential for normal growth, cell function, and immune function, and its highest concentration is in the retina. Zinc is essential for the functioning of an important antioxidant enzyme in the eye. Zinc supplementation has been found to reduce visual loss from macular degeneration.

Cautions. As mentioned earlier, excessive amounts of zinc can interfere with copper absorption, and it can cause fever, nausea, vomiting, and diarrhea. Researchers from Massachusetts General Hospital in Boston have noted that high levels of zinc *may* be linked to the development of Alzheimer's disease. That is not to say you should stop taking zinc, as it is vital to the functioning of the eye, but until we know more about the risk, I recommend that you take no more than a total of 100 mg a day from diet and supplements.

Copper 2 mg; RDA: 2 mg

Copper is important to the functioning of an antioxidant enzyme in your eye. In some cases, zinc supplementation can interfere with copper absorption, so I recommend taking a 2-mg supplement each day to guard against this effect and to provide adequate levels for proper functioning of the antioxidant enzyme in your eye.

Selenium 50 mcg; RDA: Daily Value Not Established

Selenium is similar to zinc, copper, and manganese, and is an important component of an antioxidant enzyme in your eye.

Cautions. It may cause gastrointestinal upset, but for those who can tolerate it, I recommend a 50 mcg daily supplement, in addition to dietary intake of up to 50 mcg a day.

Manganese 3.5 mg; RDA: Daily Value Not Established

This is vital to the functioning of a strong antioxidant enzyme that is present in your eye. I recommend supplementing 3.5 mg a day.

DAILY VITAMIN AND MINERAL SUPPLEMENT RECOMMENDATIONS

Nutrient (unit)	Supplement Intake
Beta-carotene (IU)	5,000
Vitamin C (mg)	1,000
Vitamin E (IU)	400
Zinc (mg)	45
Selenium (mcg)	50
Copper (mg)	2
Manganese (mg)	3.5

Multivitamins and Minerals

The table above gives you all the nutrients and minerals you need from supplements. The simplest way to get this is to find one multivitamin supplement that comes close to including all of the above nutrients, then buy supplements for the others to make up the difference. For example, if one multivitamin and mineral supplement has only 20 IU of vitamin E, then buy some additional vitamin E capsules so you can take another 380 IU each day. Also, because it is a good idea to take vitamin C several times a day rather than all at once, consider how much you need in addition to the multivitamin, and take smaller amounts at other times during the day.

There are special multivitamins designed for vision, but the vitamin E and C levels in these are too low, and most do not include manganese, so I don't recommend them. Your medical doctor may want you to take calcium, iron, and folic acid. By starting with one general multivitamin, you can add additional individual supplements to meet the requirements of other conditions and the recommendations of other physicians. If you take one supplement for your heart, one for your eyes, and one for your arthritis, the overlap may give you toxic amounts of some, such as vitamin A. Remember, too much zinc is not good either and could be implicated in Alzheimer's disease.

My own daily regimen is one multivitamin (Centrum Silver, Theragran-M, Geritol Complete, One-A-Day) and vitamin E 400 IU, vitamin C 500 mg twice a day, zinc 30 mg, and selenium 50 mcg.

Make sure your vitamins are fresh. Vitamins C and E are sensitive to both light and oxygen, and their potency diminishes with time. Always check expiration dates before buying: the regulations for vitamins are less strict than for prescription drugs. The expiration date is determined by the manufacturer. Don't buy supplements with expiration dates within six to twelve months. Look instead for dates one to two years ahead, or more.

A Word About Bilberry

Many people have asked me about bilberry as a way to restore vision to people with macular degeneration. There is no solid evidence to suggest that bilberry can help restore or preserve vision in people with macular degeneration. The small body of evidence that does exist suggests that it helps with night vision; unlike the research upon which this book is based, this research does not come from prominent universities and research centers. Until there is such evidence, I do not recommend bilberry supplements.

More Than Supplements

Never use supplements as a substitute for a healthy diet. Sometimes people rely on these and think they do not have to worry about eating their veggies or balancing their diet.

STEP 2

BEGIN A DIET RICH IN ANTIOXIDANTS AND LOW IN FAT

It is time to formulate your diet. Your main goal is to boost your antioxidants, particularly beta-carotene, lutein, and zeaxanthin, and to minimize your fat intake. Target dietary intakes for these and other antioxidants are given below. This first step in formulating your plan is to understand your overall dietary needs. Next, you will need to learn which vegetables and fruits are most nutritious, and finally you will need to know how to prepare them in the most nutritious fashion. In this section you will learn how.

NUTRIENTS YOU MUST GET FROM YOUR DIET

Vitamin/Mineral	Dietary Intake
Beta-carotene	20,000–50,000 IU
Lutein and zeaxanthin	2,500–25,000 mcg

NUTRIENTS YOU GET FROM SUPPLEMENTS AS WELL AS DIET

Vitamin/Mineral	Dietary Intake
Vitamin C	Up to 500 mg
Vitamin E	Up to 100 IU
Selenium	Up to 50 mcg
Zinc	Up to 55 mg
Manganese	Up to 5 mg
Copper	Up to 2.0 mg

7

Eat Right and See the Results

Eating the right foods for preserving your vision *and* being in the best of health means (1) maximizing your intake of antioxidants and (2) maintaining a balanced and appealing diet that meets your body's total needs, including controlling your weight. This can be done! Let's first look at the basic components of the human diet and learn why they are important.

Six to eleven servings of grains provide carbohydrates (for energy), trace minerals, and soluble and insoluble fiber (see the table on page 77 for serving sizes of grains and other food groups discussed in this section). Fiber provides bulk, and helps create the feeling of being full after a meal. Soluble fiber, also found in fruit, helps to bind certain fats in the intestine and, by preventing their absorption, helps to reduce blood cholesterol levels. Insoluble fiber is important for the digestive tract, helping to prevent constipation, diverticulosis, and colon cancer.

Vegetables (three or more servings) and fruits (two or more servings) are the basis for the dietary part of the MD Four-Step Program. Fruits and vegetables are power-houses rich in antioxidants, phytochemicals, soluble and insoluble fibers, vitamins, minerals, and other beneficial substances.

Fresh vegetables or pieces of fruit make an excellent snack: a handful of baby carrots, a half-cup of strawberries, or a medium-sized peach, for instance, will help stave off hunger *and* provide important nutrients. Don't be afraid to experiment with a variety of fruits and vegetables. You might even want to set a goal of trying a new fruit or vegetable each week.

Keep in mind that if the vegetables and fruits you eat provide a wide range of colors, you are also getting a wide range of nutrients in addition to the beta-carotene, vitamin C, lutein, and zeaxanthin, which are so important to preserving your vision.

The bottom line: Start incorporating a variety of vegetables and fruits into your daily diet. And any fruit or vegetable is better for you than a bag of potato chips!

Dairy products (2 to 3 servings)—nonfat being the best choice—are an important source of calcium needed for healthy bones. The National Institutes of Health currently recommend 1,200 mg of calcium a day for men and women on hormone replacement, and 1,500 mg for women who are not on hormone replacement, yet the typical multivitamin provides only 20 percent of calcium needs. One eight-ounce serving of fat-free milk or yogurt contains 300 mg of calcium, and most dairy products are fortified with vitamin D, which is critical to calcium absorption. Dairy products are also a good source of protein.

Proteins (2 to 3 servings of 2 or 3 ounces) along with iron, come from animal products, beans, and soy products such as tofu (tofu is also a good source of calcium). Water aside, protein is the most significant component in living matter including the human body, and makes up many of the structural elements (muscle, for example), plus enzymes, transport functions, and many others.

But there are plenty of healthy people who do not eat

meat to get their protein. Western cultures have historically used meat as the centerpiece of the meal, while Eastern cultures focus on grains and vegetables and use meat sparingly. Care is needed in the selection and preparation of animal sources of protein, as many are rich in fat, saturated fat, and cholesterol. Proteins serve an important function in the body, however, and we cannot simply eliminate them. Choose nonfat dairy products, egg substitute, fish, or low-fat meats such as skinless chicken or turkey breast. Pork producers have recently joined the health parade and are marketing meat from less fatty hogs, but don't be fooled. They still contain significantly more fat than does the white meat of turkey and chicken. If you do opt for a vegetarian diet, be sure to replace animal products with beans and legumes, tofu, or other soy products to provide the proteins you need.

Working with these five food groups, and incorporating the foods emphasized earlier that are rich in antioxidants, we can plan our meals not only for better vision, but for better overall health. But this will not just happen! To help you become an expert, there are basics to learn. The Food Guide Pyramid (figure 7.1) is an excellent place to start.

Your need to exceed these minimums will depend on your activity level and weight goals. Focus first on increasing your servings of grains, vegetables, and fruits. Remember, eating more vegetables and fruits will increase your dietary intake of antioxidants.

By exploring the recipes in Part 3, and looking at the nutritional content of different items in subsequent chapters, you will get a better idea of ways to meet your nutritional goals. And, once you are familiar with preparing food in a nutritious manner, it will be easier to create your own recipes, choose from among others, and order meals in a restaurant. Whatever you do, have fun and enjoy eating a healthy diet. Your eyes will thank you for it.

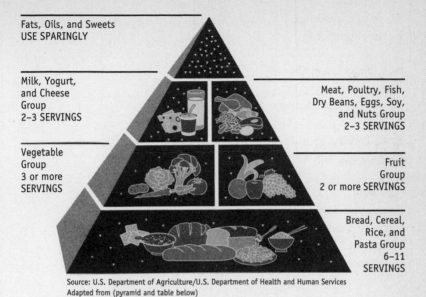

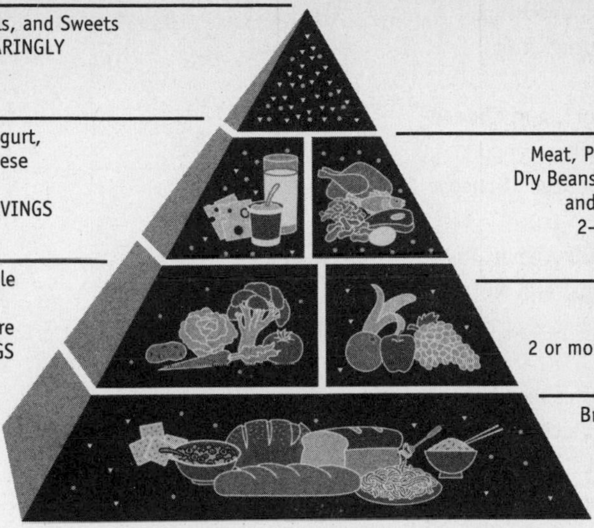

Source: U.S. Department of Agriculture/U.S. Department of Health and Human Services
Adapted from (pyramid and table below)

Figure 7.1. The Food Guide Pyramid
A Guide to Daily Food Choices

WHAT COUNTS AS ONE SERVING

Breads, Cereals, Rice, and Pasta

1 slice of bread
½ cup of cooked rice or pasta
½ cup of cooked cereal
1 ounce of ready-to-eat cereal

Vegetables

½ cup of chopped raw or cooked vegetables
1 cup of leafy raw vegetables

Fruits

1 piece of fruit or melon wedge
¾ cup of juice

½ cup of canned fruit
¼ cup of dried fruit

Milk, Yogurt, and Cheese
1 cup of milk or yogurt
1½ to 2 ounces of cheese

Meat, Poultry, Fish, Dry Beans, Eggs, and Nuts
2½ to 3 ounces of cooked lean meat, poultry, fish, or meat substitute
1½ cups of cooked beans
3 eggs or ¾ cup egg substitue
¾ cup nuts
6 tablespoons of peanut butter

8

Vegetables Ranked: Four-Star Antioxidants

You know about four-star restaurants and hotels, but some vegetables rank very high, too, especially in the antioxidants that are so important to your macula as well as your general health. To carry four stars and rank as excellent, the beta-carotene, lutein, and zeaxanthin concentration in one-half cup of the raw vegetable had to be equal to, or greater than, the minimum recommended daily intake for the MD Four-Step Program. Naturally, a half-cup of raw spinach doesn't amount to much once you wilt it or steam it, so this can be a bit misleading.

Vegetables are ranked in this chapter and fruit in the following chapter.

**** **Excellent.** To rank as excellent, the beta-carotene, lutein, and zeaxanthin concentration in a half-cup of raw vegetable had to be equal to or greater than the minimum recommended daily dietary intake for the MD Four-Step Program. For vitamin C, this ranking required a value of 250 mg, or half the recommended maximum daily dietary intake. (As we saw in chapter 6, getting this much vitamin C from your diet is difficult, and this is evident in this section as well.) The minimum recommended intake of vitamin C comes from supplements, with a target range for dietary intake of up to 500 mg per day.

*** **Good.** Three-star vegetables had to provide greater than 20 percent but less than 100 percent of the level of beta-carotene, lutein, and zeaxanthin needed for the rank of excellent, and also of the 250-mg requirement for vitamin C.

** **Fair.** For two stars, the vegetable had greater than 1 percent but less than 20 percent of these values.

* **Poor.** A one-star ranking was given for any food with less than one percent of the values required for a rank of excellent.

Where lutein and zeaxanthin are not listed, values were not available.

The four-star or excellent vegetables are the ones with the greatest nutritional value, and are the ones to concentrate on in your diet. Keep in mind that the darker the color, the higher the nutrient value. On pages 111–120 are tables separately listing the best dietary sources of each antioxidant.

If a fruit or vegetable receives only a one- or two-star rating, or is not included in the list, this does not mean you should never eat it. It just means they are not the best choices for the prevention of MD, though they may still contain a number of other beneficial nutrients.

ARTICHOKES

Artichokes are tall, rough-looking plants, of which the edible part is actually the flower bud. The petals are meaty at the base, and the artichoke heart is a great delicacy. Artichokes are best steamed then served hot or cold with a vinaigrette. Look for compact artichokes that are heavy for their size, with plump, crisp, tightly closed leaves.

** **vitamin C**
* **beta-carotene**

ARUGULA

Arugula was first used by the ancient Romans in their salads. It has small, smooth, notched leaves of dark green, and is related to the mustard family. With its spicy, tart taste and slightly bitter aftertaste, arugula is very good raw in salads mixed with other greens and accompanied by a vinaigrette or other dressing. In the south of France and in Italy, mesclun—a dish of baby mixed greens with arugula—is very popular. Arugula is higher in vitamin C than most lettuces, and rich in beta-carotene. Choose dark green leaves that are not wilted.

** **beta-carotene**
* **vitamin C**

Asparagus

Asparagus is a Eurasian plant with tender young shoots. Varieties include green, white, and purple, of which green is most common. Asparagus can be eaten cooked or raw, but is best cooked. When eaten raw, the tips are best. Asparagus is very good cooked and served cold with a vinaigrette dressing. Choose asparagus that has been kept chilled and is firm. Look for tightly closed tips that are purplish or deep green.

** **beta-carotene, vitamin C**

Bamboo Shoots

In Asian dishes, these slightly acid shoots complement mushrooms and meat. They must be young and tender; boil fresh shoots in water for ten to fifteen minutes. Fresh shoots are more nutritious than the canned type, which lose most of their vitamins and minerals.

* **beta-carotene, vitamin C**

Beans

A wide variety of beans is available, including green, wax, Italian green, lima, fava, cranberry, and black-eyed peas. As a protein-rich food, beans have nourished people of many cultures over the ages. Green beans are good raw in a salad, or cooked. They are best when firm, with well-filled pods that are not pale, do not have spots, and have lots of snap.

Green beans
*** **lutein and zeaxanthin**
** **beta-carotene, vitamin C**
Lima beans
** **beta-carotene, vitamin C**

Beets

Beets are root vegetables with a beautiful red color and a distinctive flavor. They are delicious in soups such as borscht, or served warm as a side dish. Beets are wonderful roasted. Select young, small, deep red beets that are hard, smooth, and free of bruises. The greens, which are slightly bitter, with an earthy after-taste, make an excellent dish when eaten young. Buy them young, crisp, and dark green, avoiding any that are limp. They can be eaten raw, with a light vinaigrette or other low-fat dressing, or cooked, such as lightly steamed and served with lemon juice. Beet greens are best in recipes with other vegetables.

Beets
** **vitamin C,**
* **beta-carotene, lutein, and zeaxanthin**
Beet greens
** **beta-carotene, vitamin C**

Broccoli

Broccoli is a member of the mustard family, with a spicy, peppery flavor; it is very good raw in salads or cooked. It should be kept in a cool, dry place before use. Choose broccoli with purplish or dark green florets that are tightly packed, and crisp, slender stalks. Broccoli is also thought to help prevent cancer. It is delicious served with citrus.

*** **lutein and zeaxanthin, vitamin C**
** **beta-carotene**

Brussels Sprouts

These are actually tiny cabbages. Belgians (who named them after their capital city) insisted that they be the size of a grape, and French royalty rejected any larger than a pea. Most Brussels sprouts are washed and trimmed before you purchase them. Trim off withered leaves, and the stalk. Take care not to cut the stalk too close to the base, or the leaves will fall off. Try them steamed with ginger. Fresh sprouts should be bright green, small, firm, and compact, with no wilted or blemished leaves.

*** **lutein and zeaxanthin**
** **beta-carotene, vitamin C**

Cabbage

One of the most popular vegetables in the world, cabbage is used in many different recipes. Raw or cooked, it is delicious. Varieties include green, red, purple, Savoy (which has curly leaves), or Chinese cabbage (bok choy), which has a shape more like a bunch of celery. Green cabbage is best cooked or shredded in coleslaw; red cabbage is good served raw in a mixed salad. Choose heavy cabbage heads that are solid and have only a few loose outer leaves. Avoid buying heads of cabbage that have been cut in half, as they lose a great deal of vitamin C.

Green cabbage
** **vitamin C**
* **beta-carotene**
Chinese cabbage (bok choy)
** **beta-carotene, vitamin C,**
* **lutein and zeaxanthin**
Red cabbage
** **vitamin C**
* **beta-carotene, lutein and zeaxanthin**
Savoy cabbage
** **beta-carotene, vitamin C, lutein and zeaxanthin**

Carrots

The carrot is a Eurasian plant from the parsley family. Because they are root vegetables, most people prefer to peel the bitter skin before cooking or eating. Cooking carrots until crisp but tender will increase the availability of the beta-carotene, but overcooking will decrease beta-carotene content. Like most vegetables, carrots should be kept in a chilled place to keep them fresh. Choose carrots that are dark orange, crisp, and firm, have no rootlets on their surface, and are sold in plastic, moisture-retaining packages. If you choose carrots with green tops, be sure that they are not soft and wilted.

**** **beta-carotene**
** **lutein, zeaxanthin, vitamin C**

Cassava Leaf

Cassava is a shrublike tropical plant widely grown for its large, tuberous, starchy roots, the basis for tapioca. The leaf can be eaten raw in salads or cooked (the root must be cooked before eating). Choose clean roots that are dry, hard, and have white flesh.

** **beta-carotene**

Cauliflower

The delicately flavored clustered "curds" are excellent as a hot side dish, typically with a light cream sauce. Try steaming and sprinkling lightly with dill, caraway seeds, or low-fat cheese. Cauliflower florets can also be served in salads or as a crudité. Before cooking, remove the outer leaves and most of the stem. Cauliflower should be white to creamy white with firm, compact heads free of spots. Avoid heads with open clusters or limp leaves attached.

** **vitamin C**
* **beta-carotene, lutein and zeaxanthin**

Celery

Green (i.e., unbleached) celery stalks have a higher vitamin content than their paler counterpart. Fresh celery is excellent raw in salads or as a crudité; it can also be the basis for soups. The leaves, often discarded, can be chopped and combined in omelets or added to soup stock. Select celery with crisp, compact stalks and leaf stems, with fresh green leaves. The darker green the celery, the more nutrients, but it tends to be more stringy. The greener the better.

*** **lutein and zeaxanthin**
* **beta-carotene, vitamin C**

Chicory

Chicory comes in several varieties (see curly endive). It has a slightly bitter aftertaste and is very good raw in a salad with a vinaigrette. It can also be served cooked. Look for tender, dark green leaves with a yellow center, free of discolored edges.

** **beta-carotene, vitamin C**

Chili Peppers

These peppers add a pleasant spice to many foods, and are popular in Mexican dishes, as well as some Asian and Middle Eastern foods. There are many varieties of chili, from the small green jalapeño to the larger dark purple ancho, and they are in wide use today in restaurant cooking. You can buy them fresh or powdered from most specialty stores and many markets. They should be chopped finely and added sparingly until the desired flavor is reached. Be sure not to touch your eyes after chopping—the juice can burn them! Choose peppers that are firm, have fresh green stems, and skin that is glossy and wrinkle free without soft or black spots.

*** **vitamin C**
** **beta-carotene, lutein and zeaxanthin**

Collard Greens

Collard greens also originated in Europe. These greens have a spicy flavor with a tart aftertaste. Preferably served when leaves are young, tender, and crisp, collard greens are best when cooked. They can be boiled, or braised with other vegetables. Choose moist, smooth, unwilted leaves that are dark green in color. Popular in the South, cooked with pork and fat, they are also good cooked and sprinkled with fresh lemon juice.

*** **beta-carotene**
** **vitamin C**

Corn

Purists maintain that for truly delicious corn, the ears must be steamed and served within minutes—or certainly hours—of picking. Corn can be served hot on the cob, or its kernels can be used in soups, salads, and breads. Choose yellow corn over white for greater beta-carotene content, preferably freshly picked and still in the husk. Husks should be moist and green, kernels should be plump and in tightly packed rows, and silk should be soft and golden. A kernel should pop easily when pricked with a fingernail, or the corn is probably old and tough.

Yellow corn
*** **lutein, zeaxanthin**
** **beta-carotene, vitamin C**

Cress and Watercress

Cress is not as common as watercress, but both are from the mustard family. It is grown primarily by home gardeners who appreciate its distinct flavor. It can be added to hot dishes or served in salads and sandwiches, like its cousin, watercress. Watercress has a sweet, peppery taste and has been used for both food and medicinal purposes. In the wild, it grows profusely along streams and rivers in limestone-rich areas. Watercress has smooth, round leaves and crunchy stems, and is very good mixed with other salad greens and accompanied by vinaigrette or other dressing; it can also be served in recipes, such as soup. Store watercress upright in a chilled place. Choose dark green leaves that are firm and free of spots.

Cress
** **beta-carotene**
** **vitamin C**
Watercress
** **beta-carotene**
** **vitamin C**

Cucumber

Cucumbers grow on vines, and should be harvested while young. They make an excellent addition to salads and are excellent as the basis for cold soups such as gazpacho. Buy unwaxed cucumbers, or peel them to discard the wax and any fertilizer or pesticide residue. Purchase cucumbers that are very firm and round, and that have no soft spots or shriveled tips. They range in size from the smaller Kirby cucumbers to long, slim "gourmet" cucumbers, which are generally crisper than the ordinary cucumber.

** **lutein and zeaxanthin**
* **beta-carotene, vitamin C**

Eggplant

This is one of the most versatile vegetables. The most popular variety is the large, deep purple "Black Beauty," but there are smaller varieties as well. It should be firm and evenly colored, without cuts or scars. Best when cooked, but it can also be served raw in a salad. For centuries, egg-plant was high on Europe's list of dangerous and immoral foods, but the people of the Near and Far East knew better. An eggplant should be heavy and have smooth, even-colored skin without bruises or tan patches. The deeper purple varieties will have more nutrients. There are also white ones, and small Chinese eggplants.

*** beta-carotene, vitamin C**

Endive, Belgian

The Belgian endive is the result of burying the curly endive in moist earth and keeping it in darkness. The compact head of long, thin leaves is best harvested at five to six inches long. The leaves are pale yellow and white or red and yellow, with green tips. As with curly endive, Belgian endive loses its bitterness when steamed; to help preserve its color, use a little lemon juice. It is good cooked, or raw in a salad. Choose a compact head with creamy-colored leaves that are crisp and velvety.

*** beta-carotene, vitamin C**

Endive, Curly

The curly endive family includes several types of salad greens with low-growing heads of large, frill-edged leaves. Curly endive can be eaten raw with vinaigrette or cooked in a recipe. Steaming for a few minutes removes the bitter taste. It is popular in Italian kitchens, sautéed with garlic.

**** beta-carotene**
*** vitamin C**

Fennel

Fennel is a tall, very attractive plant with a flavor like licorice. It was used by the ancient Greeks and Romans to give them strength, courage, long life, and good eyesight.

Fennel is a bulb with celerylike stalks ending in flowers that resemble dill. The entire plant is edible, raw or cooked.

Fennel leaves
** **beta-carotene, vitamin C**

Fiddlehead Fern

Fiddleheads are very young shoots of fern that grow in shady woods. The name derives from their graceful shape, curled at the top like the scroll on a fiddle. Fiddlehead ferns can be eaten raw, or cooked and chilled, with vinaigrette or other dressing. Like most greens, these are also best when young and tender. Select small fiddleheads that are bright green and tightly coiled. They are generally available during a short season in the spring.

** **beta-carotene, vitamin C**

Garlic

Garlic contains a number of nutrients for good health, and is great for adding flavor to foods. It is most nutritious raw, but the flavor is very strong. Try mincing fresh garlic and adding it to soups, sauces, and sautés. It is very good when roasted with other vegetables, or roasted and used as a spread on bread. Choose garlic bulbs that are plump and firm and have not sprouted. Always peel garlic just before using, and keep in mind that crushed garlic has three times the impact of minced garlic.

* **beta-carotene, vitamin C**

Jerusalem Artichoke

This is not an actual artichoke, nor does it come from Israel; it is the tuberous root of the North American sunflower, so named because its flavor is similar to the French artichoke. Blanched and simmered in a light sauce,

Jerusalem artichokes make an excellent accompaniment to many meat dishes. They are also called sunchokes. It is best to purchase those that are clean, firm, and have no blemishes.

* **beta-carotene, vitamin C**

Kale

Kale is a member of the mustard family with firm green and purple leaves. Because of its strong flavor and toughness, kale is best cooked and mixed with other greens. It can also be cooked and chilled, served in a mixed salad. Kale is good as a component of court bouillon soup, or used to wrap and cook fish or meat. Be sure to purchase deeply colored kale that has not wilted.

**** **lutein and zeaxanthin**
*** **beta-carotene**
** **vitamin C**

Leeks

Leeks, which resemble long, thick onions, are originally from Europe and have a strong onionlike flavor. They are easy to digest, the white part near the root being more tender than the green tops. The white part can be served in salads when steamed or poached. The green part is also good when cooked, and enhances the flavor of many dishes, particularly soups and sauces. The related green onions or scallions are popular in salads. Look for green tops that are firm, with no wilting or yellowing, and white bulbs that have no blemishes.

*** **lutein and zeaxanthin**
* **beta-carotene, vitamin C**

Lettuce

Lettuce, the basis for most salads, was first eaten in Roman times. Its many varieties include leaf, romaine, Boston, and butterhead. Fresh lettuce has green, crisp leaves. While lettuce is typically served with vinaigrette or other dressing, it can also be lightly steamed or braised. Choose the darker green or red-tinged varieties of lettuce for increased beta-carotene, vitamin C, and lutein and zeaxanthin content. Lettuces, as with all salad greens, should be fresh and crisp, with no signs of wilting or yellowing. Head lettuces, such as iceberg and radicchio, should be compact and heavy. Loose-leaf lettuces should have healthy outer leaves with no discolored tips. Iceberg is the least tasty or nutritionally valuable variety.

Iceberg
** **beta-carotene**
* **vitamin C**

Leaf
*** **lutein and zeaxanthin**
** **beta-carotene**
* **vitamin C**

Mushrooms

Low in calories, mushrooms come in many varieties for adding interest to foods. They can range in flavor from the black chanterelle, which has a musky flavor, to the richly flavored shiitake. They are good baked, sautéed, stir-fried with vegetables, and grilled as well as raw. Their meaty texture makes them a good meat substitute; try grilling a portobello mushroom and serving it on a hamburger bun.

* **beta-carotene, vitamin C, lutein and zeaxanthin**

Mustard Greens

Mustard greens are peppery and spicy, with a tart aftertaste. The entire plant is edible, leaves, stalks, and buds. Mustard greens are especially tasty and tender when the plant is young. While they can be eaten raw, they are best cooked, which gives them a milder flavor. Much like kale, these greens are good in court bouillon soup or cooked and chilled in a mixed salad. Select unwilted greens that do not have any seeds attached, as these are a sign of overmaturity.

****** lutein and zeaxanthin**
**** beta-carotene, vitamin C**

OKRA

Okra, best known as an ingredient in gumbo, has a delicate flavor, similar to eggplant. It is best when cooked, but not overcooked, which gives it a slimy texture. The best okra is young, clean, and crisp with no dark spots, bruises, or punctures.

**** beta-carotene, vitamin C**

ONIONS

Onions are low in most nutrients, but contain substances that may help you maintain a healthy heart and good circulation. They are an essential seasoning for many foods, imparting a lot of flavor with little sodium or calories. When General Grant had difficulty requisitioning them during the Civil War, he informed the War Department, "I will not move my army without onions." He got them, and this was not the only time onions were used to enliven dull army food. They vary from sweet to spicy. The Bermuda, Spanish, pearl, Vidalia, white, yellow, and red varieties are just a few that are called "dry" onions, since they do not require refrigeration. Shallots and garlic are specialty onions used for seasoning. Green onions, scallions, leeks, and chives are also onions, but perish more easily and require refrigeration. They are good raw in salad or as a garnish, as well as cooked. Almost any cooking method can be used, and they are great sliced raw on sandwiches and salads. Select onions that are solid and have no spots or sprouts.

**** vitamin C**
*** lutein and zeaxanthin, beta-carotene**

Peas

Select those with bright green, tender, slightly velvety pods. The pods should be well filled. There are new varieties of peas, such as Chinese pea pods, and snap peas, which can be eaten pod and all. Pea sprouts are also becoming popular and can be found in many gourmet markets. Use as soon as possible after buying.

***** lutein and zeaxanthin**
**** beta-carotene, vitamin C**

Pumpkin

Pumpkin is actually winter squash and can be classified as a fruit. Pumpkin has a thick orange-yellow rind and lots of seeds; it needs to be cooked to be edible, and is typically prepared as pumpkin pie, a favorite American dessert. It also makes a nutritious soup. Simply cook the pumpkin flesh, drain and puree, thin with a nonfat vegetable broth, and sprinkle on nutmeg. Choose small, firm pumpkins that are heavy and have no soft spots. Most of us get our pumpkin canned and in a pie at Thanksgiving.

***** lutein and zeaxanthin**
**** beta-carotene, vitamin C**

Scallions

See leeks, above.

Spinach

Spinach was introduced to Europe in the sixteenth century by the Moors (northern Africans) when they invaded Spain, and is now cultivated all over the world. Spinach can be eaten as a salad, preferably with a hot dressing or vinaigrette, and is also delicious cooked. Because spinach contains a lot of water, it should be blanched and drained before being included in a recipe. Or, after washing, simply chop it and add it to soup or beans that are cooking. It is particularly nice with navy or pinto beans, or black-eyed peas. For the most nutrients, spinach leaves should be small, bright green, and crisp tender, without coarse, thick stems or yellow spots on the leaves.

The nutritional value of cooked spinach is higher, not because the cooking enhances its nutritional value, but because four cups of uncooked spinach results in one-half cup of cooked spinach as a result of water loss. The half-cup of cooked spinach is denser, and contains more nutritional value, than a half-cup of raw spinach. If you were to eat the four cups of fresh spinach it took to get the half cup of cooked spinach, the four cups of raw spinach would have more nutritional value.

Raw
*** **lutein and zeaxanthin**
** **beta-carotene, vitamin C**
Cooked
**** **lutein and zeaxanthin**
*** **beta-carotene**
** **vitamin C**

SQUASH

Squash comes in many varieties, classified as either winter or summer squash. Summer squash, which includes zucchini, has sweet, meaty flesh and can be enjoyed raw as a crudité, or in salads. It can also be baked into recipes for breads, or served hot as a side dish. Winter squash is best known to us as pumpkin (see above). Try other nutritious varieties like spaghetti, acorn, and butternut. All squash should be heavy for their size and have skin that is not shriveled, bruised, or with soft spots. The deeper the color of the squash, the more beta-carotene.

*** **lutein and zeaxanthin**
** **beta-carotene, vitamin C**

Sweet or Bell Peppers

Peppers, also known as sweet or bell, come in all colors such as red and yellow or orange and purple as well as the more common green variety. Their flavor makes them good sliced or chopped in salads, or cooked in a variety of recipes. They got their name from Columbus when he discovered the West Indies. He found the natives eating red and green pods that contained all the fire of East Indian black peppers, and he called them peppers. However, botanically they are not all peppers, but come from a wider family that includes tomatoes and potatoes. Today, peppers can be lumped into two categories: sweet and hot. They are good either raw or cooked. Like chili peppers, choose sweet peppers that are firm, have fresh green stems, and skin that is glossy and wrinkle-free, without soft or black spots.

Green pepper
*** **lutein and zeaxanthin**
** **beta-carotene, vitamin C**
Red pepper
*** **vitamin C**
** **beta-carotene**

Sweet Potatoes and Yams

The sweet potato originated in the American tropics. It is a tuberous, orange-colored root with a rich, sweet taste, and is best served cooked. They are good when baked in their skin, or sliced and baked with a little orange juice. Choose sweet potatoes that are hard, smooth, heavy for their size, and with skin that is not too pale.

**** **beta-carotene**
** **vitamin C**

Swiss Chard

Swiss chard is a coarse leaf, mild in taste, from the beet family. Swiss chard can be eaten raw when the plant is young and tender, but older plants are best cooked. Choose deeply colored chard that is not wilted. Steam with garlic, or sauté. The cooked leaf is delicate, almost like spinach.

** **beta-carotene**
* **vitamin C**

Tomatoes

The tomato is classified as a fruit, but most of us consider it a vegetable. Originally from South America, it was introduced to Europe by Spanish conquistadors in the sixteenth century as a decorative plant. A century later, the Italians began using it in cooking. Tomatoes should be firm, with a bright, even color. There are twelve different varieties, and sun-dried tomatoes (available in supermarkets and health-food stores) have become popular in salads and a variety of recipes. Unlike most vegetables, some nutrients in tomatoes become more available when cooked. Tomato puree and sauce are excellent sources of beta-carotene. Choose tomatoes that are plump, heavy, and have smooth skin free of bruises. Tomatoes with soft or dark spots are beginning to deteriorate. It is best to store them at room temperature, as they are damaged by cold. Cooked tomatoes are being studied for their role in preventing prostate cancer.

Red tomato
**** **lycopene (another carotenoid antioxidant)**
** **beta-carotene, vitamin C**

Turnips and Turnip Greens

Turnips, which are root vegetables, can be braised and served as an alternative to potatoes. Turnips should be firm, smooth, and heavy for their size, while the turnip greens should be young, small, crisp, and fresh green in color. Serve mashed, with other veggies and seasonings. The greens are similar to beet greens, and can be steamed and served as an accompaniment to other vegetables.

Turnip
** **vitamin C**
* **beta-carotene, lutein and zeaxanthin**

Turnip greens, raw
** **beta-carotene, vitamin C**
* **lutein and zeaxanthin**

Turnip greens, cooked
*** **beta-carotene**
** **vitamin C**

ZUCCHINI

See squash, above.

Fresh Herbs

Many fresh herbs are an excellent source of carotenoids. Although we would not wish to eat a four-ounce serving of parsley or dill, it is helpful to remember their nutritional benefit. To maximize this, always use fresh herbs rather than dried, and add them whenever possible to salads and cooked dishes.

CILANTRO OR CORIANDER

Cilantro is generally recognized as the fresh, green plant, while coriander is the dried and ground version. It is a distinctive ingredient in many South American and Chinese recipes. It can be eaten raw or cooked, and is used primarily as a seasoning. It resembles parsley, but has a spicy citrus flavor. The leaves are oval-shaped, with serrated edges. It is a common ingredient in salsa.

** **beta-carotene**
* **vitamin C**

Dill

Dill is one of the oldest known fresh herbs. As early as 3000 B.C., the Egyptians used dill for medicinal purposes. The Greeks and Romans used it in salads for flavor; its anise-and-licorice flavor is also very good with fish and vegetables. Dill can be used raw or cooked. Because of its delicacy, it needs to be kept chilled.

*** **beta-carotene**
** **lutein and zeaxanthin**

Parsley

Parsley is one of the most common and popular fresh herbs in the world. It is believed to have the power to freshen breath after eating spicy foods. Curly parsley is generally used for decorative purposes, while the flat and aromatic Italian parsley is used in cooking. Parsley can be served either cooked or raw. It should be kept in a cool place and served while it is bright green, before it yellows.

**** **lutein and zeaxanthin**
** **beta-carotene, vitamin C**

9

Fruit Ranked: Four-Star Antioxidants

Although fruits can be an excellent source of beta-carotene and vitamin C, they are a poor source of lutein and zeaxanthin. For these nutrients, it is best to focus on green vegetables in the last chapter. As with the last chapter ranking vegetables, this glossary of fruit is ranked as excellent with four stars, good with three stars, fair with two stars, and poor with one star.

★★★★ Excellent
★★★ Good
★★ Fair
★ Poor

Just because a fruit receives a low rating or is not included on the list doesn't mean you can't eat it. It may not be the best choice for the MD Four-Step Program, but it may contain other healthful nutrients.

ACEROLA

Acerola is also known as the West Indies or Barbados cherry. Very high in vitamin C, it is used primarily as a fruit juice or in desserts or jelly. When you buy acerola, look for deep red fruit, about one inch in diameter, with a thin, smooth skin. Try blending the sweet juice with other juices for a different taste, or use the juice in a marinade for chicken, or as an ingredient in salad dressing.

**** **vitamin C**
** **beta-carotene**
As juice
**** **vitamin C**
** **beta-carotene**

APPLE

Most apples found in supermarkets are waxed to improve their appearance and retain moisture. To avoid chemical and bacterial residues trapped between the wax and the peel, peel them before you eat them. Better yet, try to find unwaxed apples (usually organically grown, or those found at farmer's markets) so you can eat the peel and get more vitamin C and beta-carotene. Look for hard, firm, well-colored apples that have been kept cold.

** **vitamin C**
* **beta-carotene, lutein and zeaxanthin**

APRICOT

Fresh apricots are a delicacy with a very short season and do not ship well. Canned or dried apricots are more available. Dried apricots are more nutritious than canned or fresh because they are a more concentrated source of nutrients, particularly beta-carotene. Canned apricots have half the vitamin C and beta-carotene of fresh ones. Fresh apricots are best eaten raw, but are also good brushed with honey and grilled as an accompaniment to fish or chicken. Dried apricots make a great snack and, when chopped, nutritious additions to cooked rice or couscous, cookies, and breads. When you do buy fresh, look for firm, plump, golden-orange apricots with velvet-smooth skin.

Fresh
** **beta-carotene, lutein and zeaxanthin, vitamin C**
Dried
*** **beta-carotene**

Banana

Bananas grow in many varieties that have somewhat different tastes and textures, but are nutritionally similar. They are most popular as a snack, but are also good mixed in a blender with other fruits and nonfat yogurt as a smoothie. Mashed or pureed, they make a great fat substitute in breads or desserts. Choose firm, unbruised bananas that are brightly colored.

** **vitamin C**
* **beta-carotene, lutein and zeaxanthin**

Blackberry

Blackberries are good on cereal and in salads and baked goods. Choose plump purplish-to-black berries that are free of mold. The darkest berries are the sweetest.

** **vitamin C**
* **beta-carotene**

Blueberry

Blueberries are a highly nutritious fruit that makes a good addition to cereals, salads, and breads. Choose berries that are plump, firm, free of mold, and deep blue with a silver-to-white shine on their surface. Discard any with red or purple skins.

** **vitamin C**
* **beta-carotene**

Cantaloupe

Cantaloupe has more beta-carotene than any other variety of melon. Select cantaloupes that are firm, golden, free of soft spots or bruises, and have a light fragrance. The stem end should be slightly indented and yield to gentle pressure.

*** **beta-carotene, vitamin C**
* **lutein and zeaxanthin**

Cherry

Fresh or dried, sour or sweet, cherries make a great snack, and are good in baking or as a base for sauces to accompany fish or chicken. Choose unbruised cherries that are firm, plump, and deep in color.

** **beta-carotene, vitamin C**

Grape

Grapes are very popular for snacking and as an addition to salads. Frozen grapes make a tasty hot-weather snack. Choose purple or red grapes over green for increased nutrient content, and look for grapes that are plump, firm, deeply colored, and have moist stems.

** **lutein and zeaxanthin**
* **beta-carotene, vitamin C**

Grapefruit

Grapefruit—pink, red, or white—provides a variety of nutrients, notably vitamin C. Choose pink or red grapefruit for increased beta-carotene, and select those that are round, firm, and feel heavy for their size.

Pink
** **beta-carotene, vitamin C**
* **lutein and zeaxanthin**

White
** **vitamin C**
* **beta-carotene, lutein and zeaxanthin**

Guava

Somewhat similar in appearance to a smooth-skinned lemon or lime, guavas are good with the seeds removed and eaten plain or as an addition to salads. Select yellow fruits that yield to gentle pressure. The pink- or red-fleshed varieties have more beta-carotene.

***** vitamin C**
**** beta-carotene**

Honeydew Melon

Honeydew is the sweetest melon variety. The flesh is usually pale green, but there are orange flesh varieties that will contain more beta-carotene. Choose honeydew that are not green but have ripened to a creamy yellow, are heavy for their size, and are free of soft or dark spots.

**** vitamin C**
*** beta-carotene, lutein and zeaxanthin**

Kiwi

Higher in vitamin C than most other fruits, kiwis are good eaten raw (the fuzzy brown skin is a good source of fiber), sliced into a fruit or dark green salad, or accompanying fish. Choose unbruised, unshriveled kiwis that are plump and yield to gentle pressure.

***** vitamin C**
*** beta-carotene, lutein and zeaxanthin**

Lemon

To add flavor to a variety of foods and beverages, choose lemons that are firm, glossy, heavy, and bright yellow. Choose fresh lemon juice for the most vitamin C.

***** vitamin C**
**** lutein and zeaxanthin**
*** beta-carotene**

Lime

Lime juice makes a good marinade for fish, and is a tasty addition to a dressing or salsa. They should be bright green in color and, like lemons, should be firm, glossy, and heavy for their size. Choose fresh lime juice over bottled or frozen for more vitamin C.

** **vitamin C**
* **beta-carotene, lutein and zeaxanthin**

Mango

Mangoes, a nutritious favorite of Indian and Caribbean cuisine, are very versatile. Try mangoes sliced with fresh lime juice squeezed over them, chunked in a fruit salad, or as a puree for desserts and in fish or chicken recipes. They are a traditional ingredient in chutney. Select mangoes that yield slightly to pressure and have an intense flowery fragrance and skins tinged with yellow-orange or red. They should not have shriveled skin or a strong smell.

** **beta-carotene, vitamin C**

Nectarine

There are a variety of nectarines, but select those with the deepest yellow or red color for the most nutrients. Try chopping them and serving over cereal, pancakes, or in a fruit salad. Choose nectarines that smell sweet, yield slightly to gentle pressure, and are free of wrinkles or bruises.

** **beta-carotene, vitamin C**

Orange

Oranges are the primary source of vitamin C for most North Americans, usually in the form of juice. Oranges make a great high-fiber snack, too, and are good in relishes and breads, and when used as a base for blender drinks. The juice makes a good marinade for fish and lean cuts of beef and chicken. Choose oranges that are smooth, firm, and feel heavy for their size. Remember that mandarin oranges have only about half as much vitamin C as other varieties.

** **beta-carotene, vitamin C**

Papaya

The papaya is a melonlike fruit filled with small, edible black seeds. It is often served grilled or chunked and sprinkled with fresh lime juice, but is also good as a puree with desserts, chicken or lean pork, or blended with other fruits as a beverage like the Apricot Divine, Sweetie Smoothie, and Hawaiian Smoothie in the recipe section. Choose firm papayas that are smooth, yellow to yellow-orange, and yield slightly to gentle pressure.

** **beta-carotene, vitamin C**
* **lutein and zeaxanthin**

Persimmon

The persimmon is a delicate fruit, very popular in Japan, and can be served baked, mashed as an accompaniment to chicken, frozen as a dessert, or cut up and served with yogurt or fruit salad. Choose persimmons that are soft, glossy, and well-rounded. Unless persimmons are very soft all over, they have a famous "puckering" effect on the mucous membranes of the mouth.

*** **beta-carotene, vitamin C**
* **lutein and zeaxanthin**

Peach

The peach is a very popular and versatile fruit, with a sweet flesh that ranges in color from white to yellow-orange. Choose the more deeply colored flesh for the most vitamin C and beta-carotene. Also check that they are firm, free of wrinkles and blemishes, smell mildly sweet, and have creamy yellow skin tinged with pink or red. Dried peaches are great as a take-along snack; also try chopping them to top a salad or to mix in muffin or bread batter.

Fresh
** **beta-carotene, vitamin C**
* **lutein and zeaxanthin**
Dried
** **beta-carotene, vitamin C, lutein and zeaxanthin**

Pear

Buy unwaxed pears and eat raw with the skin, since that is where most of the vitamin C is. Look for firm pears with smooth skin that yields slightly to pressure at the stem.

** **vitamin C, lutein and zeaxanthin**
* **beta-carotene**

Pineapple

Most often eaten fresh, pineapple is also good baked or grilled. For a novel pizza topping, use fresh broccoli, mushrooms, and pineapple chunks (don't try this in New York!) or add chunks to a stir-fry. Choose large, fresh pineapple that is firm, plump, heavy, and has fresh green leaves.

** **vitamin C**
* **beta-carotene, lutein and zeaxanthin**

Plum

There are a variety of plums, large and small, ranging from sweet to tart in flavor. Eat them fresh and whole, sliced with nonfat yogurt, or chopped and added to a green salad.

Choose deeply colored plums that are plump, unwrinkled, and yield to gentle pressure.

** **beta-carotene, vitamin C**
* **lutein and zeaxanthin**

Pomegranate

Pomegranates are a real treat! About the size of a large orange, they have thin, leathery skin that ranges from red to blushed yellow. Choose pomegranates that are brightly colored and blemish-free, and feel heavy for their size. They are filled with hundreds of tiny edible seeds, each surrounded by an edible, sweet-tart red pulp; but don't eat the bitter, cream-colored membranes. The seeds are delicious eaten alone, combined with other fruits in a fruit salad, or sprinkled on top of nonfat yogurt or ice cream.

** **vitamin C, lutein and zeaxanthin**
* **beta-carotene**

Raspberry

Raspberries are very delicate and seasonal. The red raspberry is most familiar, but there are also pale yellow and amber varieties. Raspberries make a fabulous addition to a number of foods: toss some in a bowl of cereal or yogurt or on a green salad; puree as a sauce for desserts, fish, or chicken; or drop a few in a glass of champagne for a special touch. Choose raspberries that are well colored, firm, and free of mold. Use them immediately.

** **vitamin C, lutein and zeaxanthin**
* **beta-carotene**

Star Fruit (Carambola)

Star Fruit is a slightly tart fruit that when sliced crosswise produces sections in the shape of a five-pointed star. Their unique shape makes them an excellent garnish for desserts, grain dishes, and entrees, and they are a great addition to a spinach salad. Choose well-shaped fruit that is shiny, golden yellow, and free of blemishes.

** **beta-carotene, vitamin C**

Strawberry

The most popular berry, strawberries are also the highest in vitamin C content. Strawberries' sweet flavor and bright color lend them to a wide variety of uses, most commonly as dessert. For a healthier dessert, try them with low-fat vanilla yogurt instead of whipped cream, or splashed with a little Grand Marnier liqueur or balsamic vinegar. They are another fruit that is good on a spinach salad. Choose the deepest red strawberries for the most nutrients, and select those that are firm but not hard, and are free of bruises or white spots.

** **vitamin C, lutein and zeaxanthin**
* **beta-carotene**

Tangerine

Tangerines are a type of orange. Best sectioned, seeded, and eaten fresh, they, too, are a nice addition to a dark green salad, perhaps with a citrus vinaigrette. Choose tangerines that are smooth-skinned and heavy for their size.

* **beta-carotene**
* **vitamin C, lutein and zeaxanthin**

Watermelon

Not just a picnic food, try cutting watermelon into chunks for a fruit salad, or seeding, pureeing, and freezing as an icy dessert. Choose whole watermelons that are uniformly shaped, are very heavy for their size, have a yellowish underside, and are free of soft spots.

** **beta-carotene, vitamin C**
* **lutein and zeaxanthin**

For information about how to select, store, and prepare fruits and vegetables for maximum nutrient value, see chapter 13.

10

Common Food Sources of Beta-carotene, Lutein, and Zeaxanthin

In this chapter you will find alphabetical lists of common vegetables and fruits that are good sources of beta-carotene and lutein and zeaxanthin. Since these are the three antioxidants for which you must get your minimum daily requirements from your diet, you will want to pay particular attention to this chapter.

Beta-carotene

There are many ways to use foods rich in beta-carotene. Try adding shredded carrots to a pita shell filled with sliced tomatoes, sprouts, cucumber, and fat-free cheese, or to a muffin or quick-bread batter. Add chopped dried apricots or peaches to couscous or rice, moisten with orange juice and warm. Top a microwaved sweet potato with black beans, salsa, and fat-free sour cream. And you can add chopped fresh spinach to soups, beans, or rice, or use as a pizza topping.

Your goal is to obtain at least 20,000 IU of beta-carotene per day from your diet. Since beta-carotene is converted to vitamin A, the RDA is essentially the same. Here are some possibilities:

- ¾ cup or 1½ medium-sized carrots
- ½ cup mashed sweet potatoes (1 medium-sized)
- ½ cup of dried apricots
- 1 cup of dried peaches
- 1 large baked sweet potato
- 1¼ cup cooked spinach
- 2½ cups of sliced cantaloupe

We need some fat to absorb these, because beta-carotene is fat-soluble. Most diets, even those low in fat, provide enough fat for absorption, but adding a half-teaspoon of olive oil will boost your vitamin E intake.

BETA-CAROTENE CONTENT OF COMMON FOODS
(Your goal is to get 20,000–50,000 IU per day from your diet.)

This table lists the beta-carotene content of foods for a more detailed study. Content is given in IU (international units), and to make it easy to compare the nutritional value of different foods, the beta-carotene concentration is given in half-cup portions. For leafy vegetables, this means a well-packed half-cup. For fruits or solid vegetables, it means one-half cup finely chopped. "Raw" means fresh, not dried, canned, or cooked. For accuracy, the measurements are given as "finely chopped," but to maximize the nutritional content, it is best to use larger rather than smaller pieces for food preparation.

Food	Beta-carotene (IU)	Calories per ½ cup	Oz. per ½ cup
Apricot, canned, drained	2,841	25	4.0
Apricot, raw	4,504	37	2.7
Apricot, dried	19,166	155	2.3
Beet greens, cooked	3,030	20	2.5
Broccoli, cooked	1,693	22	2.75
Broccoli, raw	514	12	1.55
Cantaloupe, raw	3,977	28	2.8

Food	Beta-carotene (IU)	Calories per ½ cup	Oz. per ½ cup
Carrot, raw	16,763	24	1.94
Carrot, cooked	33,399	35	2.75
Celery, raw, diced	713	10	2.12
Chicory leaf, raw	6,248	21	3.18
Coriander, not dried	267	2	0.28
Cress leaf, raw	1,733	8	0.88
Endive	543	4	0.88
Fennel leaves	496	4	0.50
Grapefruit, pink, raw	2,518	35	4.06
Green beans	656	22	2.20
Greens, collard, boiled	8,565	26	3.35
Greens, collard, raw	1,636	6	0.64
Greens, fiddlehead, boiled	1,440	9	1.56
Greens, mustard, cooked	3,132	11	2.45
Greens, mustard, raw	1,266	7	0.99
Guava, raw	1,115	42	2.90
Kale, cooked	5,100	21	2.29
Kale, raw	2,626	17	1.18
Leek, raw	743	27	1.57
Lettuce, leaf	561	5	0.98
Lettuce, romaine	898	5	0.98
Mango, raw	1,791	54	2.91
Mushroom, chanterelle, raw	757	9	1.23
Parsley, not dried	2,685	11	1.07
Peach, dried	12,271	191	2.80
Pepper, red	2,729	20	2.62
Pumpkin, canned	6,341	42	4.32
Scallion, raw	708	16	1.76
Spinach, cooked, drained	8,268	21	3.17
Spinach, raw	1,027	3	0.52
Squash, winter, cooked	4,109	40	3.60
Squash, winter, raw	797	21	2.05
Sweet potato, mashed	24,167	172	5.80
Sweet potato, baked	14,584	103	3.50
Sweet potato, raw	9,886	70	2.35

Food	Beta-carotene (IU)	Calories per ½ cup	Oz. per ½ cup
Tomato, raw	781	19	3.18
Tomato juice, canned	1,834	21	4.30
Tomato paste, canned	465	13	0.58

Lutein and Zeaxanthin

The easiest and best way to get the 2,500 mg of lutein and zeaxanthin you need from your diet each day is to eat a mixed salad of spinach and leafy lettuce, one cup twice a day, or snack on a stalk of celery every day. Spinach has the highest concentration of lutein and zeaxanthin, but other green leafy vegetables such as kale and collard greens are high. Celery, broccoli, dill, leek, green peas, romaine lettuce, pumpkin, and summer squash also contain these nutrients.

You can incorporate lutein and zeaxanthin into your diet by adding fresh chopped parsley, dill, or spinach to add flavor and nutrients to cold salads or cooked foods. Small amounts will add up! Also, try snacking on celery sticks filled with a fat-free herb dip, or eating sautéed spinach or other dark greens splashed with raspberry vinegar or balsamic vinegar. Green peas are excellent eaten cold on a green salad, or as an addition to a pasta salad made with fresh chopped broccoli, red peppers, carrots, and a fat-free Italian dressing or other vinaigrette.

Here's what you need to get your daily 2,500-mg requirement:

- 1 cup of cooked broccoli (approximately one large spear)
- ⅛ cup cooked spinach
- ¼ cup cooked mustard greens
- ⅛ cup cooked kale
- 1 cup green peas

Remember, spinach and other leafy vegetables shrink when cooked because they contain large amounts of water.

As you will learn in chapter 13, proper storage and preparation of these foods is vital to preserve the nutritional content.

LUTEIN AND ZEAXANTHIN CONTENT OF COMMON FOODS
(Your goal is to get 2,500–25,000 mcg per day from your diet.)

Nutritionists have only just begun to examine the lutein and zeaxanthin levels in vegetables and fruits, so values are not available for many of them.

Food	Lutein and zeaxanthin, mcg per ½ cup	Calories per ½ cup	Oz. per ½ cup
Avocado	367	129	4.05
Beets (cooked)	3.4	17	0.99
Broccoli (raw)	836	12	1.55
Broccoli (cooked)	1,404	22	2.75
Brussels sprouts	572	30	1.55
Cabbage, Chinese	14	5	1.23
Cabbage, red	9	9	1.23
Cabbage, Savoy	53	9	1.23
Carrots (raw)	143	24	1.94
Cauliflower (raw)	17	13	1.76
Celery (raw)	2,160	10	2.12
Chili peppers	137	14	2.64
Corn (cooked)	640	66	2.89
Cucumber (pickle)	398	14	2.73
Cucumber (raw)	125	7	1.83
Dill, fresh, not dried	299	2	0.15
Green beans	465	22	2.20
Greens, mustard (raw)	2,784	7	0.99
Greens, mustard (cooked)	5,434	11	2.47
Kale	7,351	17	1.18
Kiwifruit, raw	160	54	3.12
Leeks (raw)	865	27	1.57
Lettuce (leaf)	504	5	1.00

Food	**Lutein and zeaxanthin, mcg per ½ cup**	**Calories per ½ cup**	**Oz. per ½ cup**
Olive, green	379	86	2.60
Onions (raw)	13	30	2.82
Parsley, not dried	2,898	11	1.00
Pear, raw	91	49	2.90
Peas	1,352	67	2.80
Pepper (green)	522	20	2.63
Pepper, yellow	572	20	2.62
Pumpkin (cooked)	863	42	2.00
Raspberries, raw	47	30	2.17
Scallions, raw	1,049	17	1.76
Spinach (raw)	1,533	3	0.53
Spinach (cooked)	11,365	21	3.17
Squash, summer (zucchini)	678	8	2.00
Tomato, raw	90	19	3.18

11

Common Food Sources of Vitamins C and E

To make it easy for you to add plenty of these important antioxidants to your diet, I have listed the food sources alphabetically in a table of the vitamin and calorie content of each. The same format is used for vitamin E, which follows the vitamin C listings.

Food Sources of Vitamin C

In order to preserve your vision you will need to get at least 1,000 mg of vitamin C daily. To get this much vitamin C from your diet alone is very difficult. As a result, my recommendation is to get the bulk of your vitamin C through a 1,000 mg daily supplement, and to augment your vitamin C intake by up to 500 mg per day by selecting items from the following list of foods with high concentrations of vitamin C. The table gives quantities in milligrams (mg) and the list is confined to fruits and vegetables because, like beta-carotene, that is where vitamin C is mostly found.

VITAMIN C CONTENT OF COMMON FOODS
(Your goal is to get up to 500 mg per day from your diet.)

Food	Vitamin C (mg)	Calories per ½ cup	Oz. per ½ cup
Acerola, trimmed	822	16	1.73
Acerola, juice	1,936	25	4.27
Acorn squash	11	58	3.62
Apricot, raw	8	37	2.73
Artichoke, hearts, boiled	8	42	2.96
Artichoke, boiled, drained	4	38	2.96
Banana	7	69	2.65
Beet greens, raw	6	7	0.67
Blackberries	15	37	2.54
Broccoli, raw	41	12	1.55
Brussels sprouts, boiled	48	44	1.55
Cabbage, raw, shredded	11	9	1.24
Cabbage, shredded, cooked	15	17	2.65
Cantaloupe	34	28	2.80
Cauliflower, fresh	36	17	1.76
Grapefruit, juice, fresh	47	48	4.36
Grapefruit, raw, sections	40	35	4.06
Guava, common	151	42	2.90
Kale, raw, chopped	40	17	1.18
Kiwifruit	87	54	3.12
Mango	23	54	2.91
Orange, California navel	47	38	2.91
Orange juice, fresh	62	56	4.37
Papaya	43	27	2.47
Pepper, sweet (bell), green	67	20	2.62
Pepper, sweet (bell), red	67	20	2.62
Potato, with skin, baked	9	74	2.15
Raspberries, fresh	15	30	2.17
Strawberries, fresh, whole	41	22	2.54
Tangerine, fresh	30	43	3.44
Tomato, fresh, diced	17	19	3.18
Watermelon, fresh	7	24	2.68

Food Sources of Vitamin E

The current RDA for this vitamin—10 IU for men and 8 for women—is probably much too low to offer much protection from oxidation. Early research has shown us that between 100 IU and 400 IU a day may be more like it. Vitamin E is relatively low in toxicity up to 800 IU a day, but if you take anticoagulants, you should not take this much.

The best sources of vitamin E include vegetable oils and seeds or nuts, such as wheat germ oil, sunflower seeds, almonds, and sunflower oil, all high in fat and calories. To get the 400–500 IU of vitamin E you need from your diet, even from the best source of natural vitamin E, you would have to consume three-quarters of a cup of wheat-germ oil or about four cups of sunflower seeds. This would amount to over 1,400 calories for the wheat-germ oil and over 3,000 calories for the sunflower seeds—more than the recommended daily calorie consumption for most people. This is obviously excessive, except for professional and endurance athletes, who can easily require 5,000 to 10,000 calories a day, but it is not recommended.

Instead, I recommend getting most of your vitamin E in the form of a 400 IU supplement, and up to another 100 IU from your diet. Because the 400 IU supplement covers your basic needs, any additional is a plus when it can be done in a calorie- and health-conscious way. For example, use olive or canola oils rich in vitamin E to cook with and for salad dressing. Wheat germ is good sprinkled over your breakfast cereal or yogurt. It is also more healthful to eat whole wheat bread, rolls, cereals, and pasta rather than refined white varieties. The whole wheat varieties contain more vitamin E, and also provide necessary fiber to the diet.

Beyond this, I do not recommend trying to increase your consumption of these foods because the benefit of the increased vitamin E is far outweighed by the downside of the extra calories and fat.

The vitamin E content of common foods is given in one-half-cup portions, as well as one-tablespoon portions. This is done because you are far more likely to use one-tablespoon portions than half-cup portions, which makes the second table more useful. Because one-half-cup values are given for the other antioxidants, they are provided for vitamin E as well.

VITAMIN E CONTENT OF COMMON FOODS
(Your goal is to get up to 100 IU per day from your diet.)

Food	Vitamin E (IU) per ½ cup	Calories per ½ cup	Oz. per ½ cup
Almonds, dry-roasted	26	405	2.43
Canola oil	35	962	3.84
Corn oil	35	962	3.84
Flax oil	29	959	3.83
Hazelnuts	20.5	396	2.38
Olive oil	20	952	3.81
Peanut butter	18.6	751	4.52
Pecans	3	360	1.91
Product 19® cereal	15	55	0.53
Safflower oil	56	962	3.84
Sunflower oil	73.5	962	3.84
Sunflower seeds	54	411	2.54
Total® cereal	24	74	0.71
Wheat germ	9	400	2.00
Wheat germ oil	314	961	3.84

	Vitamin E (IU) per tablespoon	Calories per tablespoon	Oz. per tablespoon
Canola oil	4.3	120	0.48
Corn oil	4.3	120	0.48
Flax oil	3.6	125	0.50
Olive oil	2.5	119	0.48
Peanut butter	2.3	94	0.56

	Vitamin E (IU) per tablespoon	Calories per tablespoon	Oz. per tablespoon
Safflower oil	7	120	0.48
Sunflower oil	9	120	0.48
Wheat germ	1	50	0.25
Wheat germ oil	39	120	0.48

12

Common Food Sources of Zinc and Other Minerals

Common foods rich in zinc are listed below to help you maximize zinc intake in your diet. The values for fruits and vegetables are given in one-half-cup portions, as in the other tables. Because most meat and fish is purchased by the pound, the values are given in quarter-pound (four-ounce) portions. After cooking, four ounces of meat, fish, or poultry is reduced to three ounces, which is equal to the recommended portion for one serving of protein.

ZINC CONTENT OF COMMON FOODS
(Your goal is to get up to 55 mg per day.)

Food	Zinc (mg) per ½ cup	Calories per ½ cup	Oz. per ½ cup
Avocado	0.5	129	4.05
Baked beans	1.78	118	4.48
Buckwheat flour	1.87	201	2.12
Cashew nuts, dry-roasted	3.83	393	2.41
Oats, whole grain	3.1	304	2.75
Product 19® cereal	7.5	55	0.53

Food	Zinc (mg) per ½ cup	Calories per ½ cup	Oz. per ½ cup
Raspberries	0.28	30	2.17
Spinach, raw	0.1	3	0.53
Tofu, firm	1.98	183	4.44
Yogurt, low-fat	1.1	78	4.32

	Zinc (mg) per 4 ounces	Calories per 4 ounces
Beef, ground, baked	7.87	280
Beef, sirloin, lean	8.0	193
Chicken, with skin	2.44	265
Clams, raw	1.56	84
Crayfish, boiled or steamed	1.68	99
Duck, domestic, roasted	2.10	382
Ham, fresh, roasted	2.92	223
Lamb, cubed for stew	5.97	233
Liver, calf's, pan-fried	8.92	187
Lobster, steamed	3.31	111
Oysters	42.85	67
Pork, loin, braised	2.96	297
Salmon, canned	1.16	157
Turkey, with skin	3.58	232
Veal, meat only	4.64	191

Keep in mind that zinc levels can be depressed by certain conditions, or by medications such as oral contraceptives and hormones. If you are a diabetic with retinal damage, you have less zinc than others. Read chapter 4 for more information about zinc and other minerals from supplements and foods.

Copper

You need 2 to 4 mg of copper a day for a high antioxidant diet because some of the copper in your body will be diminished by the increased amounts of vitamin C and zinc. Copper is present in many foods, but not in significant amounts to make a difference in your diet, which is why you need to meet your 2 mg minimum daily requirement in the form of a supplement. The best sources of copper are nuts and dried beans and lentils. Whole grains, raisins, and shrimp and other shellfish are good sources. In addition to your daily supplement with copper, here are the best food sources. As you can tell, the amounts are not high, and you would need to eat quite a bit of these foods to get 2 mg.

COPPER CONTENT OF COMMON FOODS
(Your goal is to get up to 2.0 mg per day.)

Food	Mg of copper per ½ cup serving
Black beans, cooked	.25
Cashews, dry-roasted	1.26
Hummus	.28
Lentils, boiled	.25
Navy beans, boiled	.27
Pasta, whole wheat, cooked	.12
Peanuts, dry-roasted	.38
Peanuts, raw	.64
Raisins, seedless	.23
Red kidney beans, canned	.19

Food	Mg of copper per 3 oz. serving
Crab, Alaska king, cooked	.10
Oysters, cooked	.23
Shrimp, cooked (15 large)	.16

SELENIUM

Selenium is found in many foods, but the best sources are whole grains and seafood. You need to get up to 50 mcg a day from food and the rest from supplements.

Here are some of the best sources:

SELENIUM CONTENT OF COMMON FOODS
(Your goal is to get up to 50 mcg per day.)

Food	Mcg of selenium per ½ cup serving
Brown rice, cooked	40
Cheerios® dry cereal	5
Cream of Wheat, cooked	19
Oatmeal, cooked	10
Tofu	11.1
Whole wheat bread, 1 slice	8.5

Food	Mcg of selenium per 3 oz. serving
Crab, blue, cooked	24
Flounder	50
Salmon, pink, canned	28
Shrimp (15 large)	40
Tuna, light, canned in water	68.5

Manganese

Manganese is poorly absorbed in the intestine, so it is important to get the recommended amount. The FDA has not established an RDA for manganese; 2 to 8.5 mg a day is a safe and adequate intake for adults. A supplement should provide about 3.5 mg, and the rest can come from food. Nuts, whole grains, and leafy vegetables are the best sources.

MANGANESE CONTENT OF COMMON FOODS
(Your goal is to get up to 5 mg per day.)

Food	Mg of manganese per ½ cup serving
Almonds	.04
Bran flakes	.85
Broccoli, raw	.01

Food	Mg of manganese per ½ cup serving
Brown rice, cooked	.89
Kale, cooked	.27
Leaf lettuce, raw	.02
Peanuts, dry-roasted	1.52
Pecans, raw	2.4
Spinach, raw	.02

13

How to Buy, Store, and Prepare Vegetables and Fruit for Maximum Nutrition

When I first learned about the vision-related benefits of eating green leafy vegetables such as spinach, collard greens, and kale, these vegetables were not a standard part of my diet. I was not sure how to prepare them, how to store them, or even whether they were better raw or cooked. My food awareness has since grown, and I have discovered these vegetables are a big part of the more dynamic and ethnically diverse cuisine that is appearing in restaurants everywhere. Today, with our increasing awareness of healthful lifestyles, vegetables and fruit are in high demand. Farmer's markets and fresh produce stands have proliferated. Nevertheless, we need to know that produce can be high or low in antioxidants and other nutrients depending on where it is grown, on weather conditions, and on how it is shipped, stored, and processed.

When you shop for fresh fruit and vegetables, shop the way you would for fine wine. In selecting a bottle of wine, you must consider a number of factors such as the type of wine, the vineyard, the year the grapes were grown, how it was stored, and how long it was stored. Similar factors affect antioxidants and other nutrients in your produce. The fact that wine quality varies with the vineyard demonstrates that the soil, the grape, and the processing are important factors. The difference in years reflects the importance of weather conditions, such as temperature, rainfall, sun, and the harvest time. The way wine is stored is critically important, as it is for produce on its way to market. And, finally, the age of the wine is important. If it is too young, its flavor may have not peaked, and if too old, it may have turned to vinegar. Thc same is true for produce.

Growing conditions can account for a 20-percent variation in vitamin C content. For example, the oranges on the south side of a tree may have more vitamin C because they were exposed to more sun. Sugar content in tomatoes is higher when the solar radiation is highest, from June to August. Tests showed that vitamin C content of carrots was highest in Seattle and Minneapolis, but that carrots grown in Atlanta fared best in carotene content.

Nutritional value can also be lost in harvesting, packing, storage, preparation, and cooking. A vegetable picked garden-fresh and frozen may have more value than produce that has been ten days in transport and two or three days in the store. For example, researchers found that harvest-fresh peas had a vitamin C content of 121 percent, canned had 102 percent, frozen had 98 percent, and market-fresh had only 65 percent.

Antioxidants are very sensitive to a number of variables in this process, including the following:

- Early harvest before the produce is ripe—common with stores.
- Exposure to oxygen, metal, light, and heat.
- Washing and soaking in water.
- Boiling in excessive amounts of water.
- Overcooking.

So here are some general guidelines for keeping your veggies full of nutrients, especially those critically important antioxidants.

Buy Garden-Fresh

Whenever you can, buy vegetables and fruits at a farmer's market or pick them from your garden. The riper the produce, and the sooner it is eaten, the more nutritious, and tasty. Much of the produce that is sold around America is picked before it is ripe and shipped across the country in trucks where the produce is treated with special gases that ripen it while it travels. Carrots harvested earlier contain less carotene than those picked later. Fresh spinach is usually four to thirteen days old before it reaches you, and can lose as much as 90 percent of its nutrients.

Farmer's markets are now in most metropolitan areas in all parts of the country, at least during the summer and fall. In some states in the South and West where produce is grown, such markets are available year-round. Once you get used to the flavor and consistency of just-picked produce, you will find it difficult to eat anything else. Fruits and vegetables with the deepest colors generally contain the highest levels of antioxidants.

"Certified" Organic Produce

Increased environmental concern has made consumers more selective, demanding food that is not contaminated with an overabundance of pesticides and fertilizer chemicals. Organic produce markets are opening around the country, and most major supermarket chains now carry organic produce as well. Twenty years ago the organic produce market consisted of a few shriveled and overpriced carrots in a health-food store.

You can now find organic produce at many large supermarket chains (especially in large metropolitan areas) as well as in specialty and gourmet food stores and farmer's markets. Organic produce is generally fresher and more nutritious than chemically treated produce. However, do not select organic produce just because it is organic. Fresh-looking, traditionally grown broccoli, for example, would be a more nutritious choice than organic broccoli with florets that are beginning to yellow.

When Fresh Produce Is Not Available

Frozen

If fresh is not available, buy frozen produce because it is picked at the peak of maturity and processed immediately. Frozen produce can be higher in nutrients than produce that has been shipped a long distance and stored for a long time. Frozen spinach is particularly good, as the loss of vitamin C in fresh spinach between harvest and market has been estimated to be as high as 90 percent.

Vegetables lose about 25 percent of their nutrients during the entire freezing process. In six months or a year, they lose another 50 percent. Once the vegetables are cooked after freezing, they lose more nutrients.

Nutrient loss during frozen storage increases with the length of time, from 10 to 20 percent for three months up to 30 to 60 percent for a year. The amount of loss is also increased if the freezer temperature is too high.

Most conventional fruits, when frozen, lose less than 30 percent of their original vitamin C, except for citrus fruits, which lose less than 5 percent. Most of this loss occurs during frozen storage. Interestingly, however, when citrus is stored in a metal can, it loses much less than when stored in cardboard—which is the way most frozen concentrated orange juice is sold.

Canned

While fresh or frozen is usually the best choice—certainly the most appealing to the eye—canned vegetables and fruit can sometimes be a good option. There is not always a significant nutritional difference when you consider the loss that some fresh produce has while being shipped and stored for long periods. The high heat in the canning process can lead to greater loss of vitamin C and the B vitamins, and softer produce. The biggest drawback of canned vegetables is that they may contain high amounts of salt, so always choose varieties without added salt or sodium.

Tomatoes are an example of a vegetable that is often superior canned, or processed into juice. This way it often contains more lycopene, a powerful antioxidant, than fresh tomatoes.

When you buy canned vegetables such as corn, many of the vitamins will be in the water that is usually discarded. Consider saving this water for cooking vegetables, or for use in broth.

Dehydrated

Sun-dried tomatoes are very popular now, but they may have only half the nutrients of fresh or canned. However, you tend to eat more of them because even after they are restored with warm water, they are smaller than fresh or canned. Sun-dried tomatoes are good with olive oil, garlic, and (low-fat) mozzarella cheese for a tasty appetizer. Most produce is dried in the sun or freeze-dried, which is the best for preserving the nutrients.

As the water is removed from the vegetable or fruit during dehydration, the concentration of nutrients increases, but they break down faster. Half the value of water-soluble vitamins like C are lost during the process. Fat-soluble vitamins degrade by a free-radical oxidation mechanism. For freeze-dried carrots, researchers reported a 13-percent loss of beta-carotene, and another study reported a 4-percent loss in freeze-dried orange juice.

Storing to Preserve Freshness

Refrigerate fresh fruits and vegetables in perforated plastic bags. The humid air of the refrigerator crisper drawer is perfectly suited to green leafy vegetables. Keep your refrigerator between 3–4.5° Celsius (37–40° Fahrenheit).

Keep your freezer temperature low—below –18° Celsius (0° Fahrenheit), but don't keep frozen foods longer than three months. The most stable foods to freeze are orange juice, green peas, cooked spinach, raspberries, strawberries, and cauliflower. If you freeze your own foods, cut them in large pieces for greater retention of nutrients. Don't thaw frozen vegetables before they are cooked.

For room-temperature storage of potatoes, onions, and unripened fruit, choose a cool, dark place. Don't sit a bowl of pears in front of a well-lighted window and expect them to maintain their nutrients for very long.

Preparation

- Don't rinse produce until you are ready to use it, or you will wash away some of the nutrients.
- Don't soak produce, or many nutrients will leach out. Many people like to scrub their vegetables in diluted soap and water to remove any possible chemical residue from pesticides or fertilizers. If you do use soap, be sure to rinse well.
- Wash green leafy vegetables under running water. When they have lots of sand embedded within the leaves, you will need to immerse them in water, but don't leave them there. Change the water a few times and shake out the leaves until the sand remains in the sink or bowl.
- Don't trim, chop, dice, or slice until you are ready to serve the food.

Cooking

Cook vegetables as little as possible to maximize their nutritional content. Excess heat and long cooking times can reduce nutrient content by as much as half—not to mention taste and texture. Microwaving or steaming preserves the nutritional content better than boiling.

Boil with as little water as possible, and in a pot with a tight-fitting lid. This will keep nutrient loss in the cooking water. Add a little lemon juice to the water before boiling to help preserve the color of greens. Keep the water from flavorful vegetables such as carrots in the freezer for use in soups and sauces.

Blanch vegetables until just tender by dropping them into a large pot of rapidly boiling water for a few minutes without a lid. Remove the vegetables and immediately plunge them into an ice bath—a bowl of ice-cold water—to stop the cooking process. This will help keep vegetables green and high in chlorophyll.

Steam vegetables by placing them in a steamer basket, placing the basket in a pot with a small amount of boiling water, and covering. Steaming for a short period of time, until vegetables are just crisp-tender, will minimize nutrient loss. To maximize nutrient retention, steam foods in the microwave using a microwave steamer.

Wilt a bunch of spinach or other greens by placing them in a shallow pan with only the water that adheres to the leaves after rinsing. Turn the heat on for a few seconds until the leaves wilt. This is a way to make green leafy vegetables just tender and warm. Another way to wilt delicate greens is to toss them with a hot salad dressing.

Braise the heavier greens such as collards for a few minutes on top of the stove. This is like taking wilting one more step. Heat the pan with a bit of olive oil, or nonfat cooking spray, sauté the vegetables for a few minutes, add a bit of liquid, such as vegetable or chicken stock, and cook covered for a few more minutes.

Microwave at the highest power and shortest cooking time. For example, you can microwave carrots for a few minutes (prick them with a fork first so they don't explode) and they will be softer than raw, but tastier and more nutritious than boiled.

Bake sweet potatoes for more taste than boiling. While baking usually destroys most of the vitamin C in any food, fat-soluble vitamins like the beta-carotene in sweet potatoes are more likely to stand up to the heat of baking. Microwave "baking" of potatoes will minimize nutrient loss.

Roast a pan of high-antioxidant vegetables like red and green peppers, garlic, onions, and squash, but try reducing the roasting time by half and finish cooking in the microwave until tender. This will save more of the nutrients.

Grill over a lower flame to reduce charring, and never eat anything that has been burned black. Grilling is easy and imparts a special flavor to foods. However, the charred appearance associated with foods off the grill is also associated with increased cancer risk.

Eat your meals as soon as they are prepared, and avoid warming for more than thirty minutes. Try using leftover vegetables in cold salads the next day so you don't have to reheat them. Nutritional content is damaged by heat, so try to avoid lengthy warming of food. Also, reheating previously cooked food further reduces its value. Vitamin C in produce is particularly susceptible to nutrient loss during warming or reheating.

14

Trimming the Fat: Low-Fat Alternatives

Fat has more than twice as many calories as either proteins or carbohydrates—nine calories per gram—whereas proteins and carbohydrates have four calories per gram. Most Americans get 40 percent of their calories from fat, but you should reduce that to no more than 20 percent. It is quite easy to eat this much fat without even being aware of it. For example, you may think a big bran muffin is a healthful breakfast item, but most muffins are baked with eggs and oil or butter—and they are generally high in fat. Packaged crackers and other snack foods are high in fats. French fries, hamburgers, and other fast foods are loaded with fat. Regular milk has plenty of fat, while skim milk has no fat but all of the nutrients.

Most of the fat you eat comes from three sources: animal products (including meats, poultry, and dairy products such as whole milk and cheeses), oils (including margarine and salad dressings), and processed foods. Processed foods include potato chips and other snack-type chips, crackers, cookies, pastries, packaged convenience entrees, and side dishes such as instant rice and pasta mixes, and other packaged snack foods.

By reducing your fat intake, you not only reduce your

risk of developing macular degeneration, but you can also reduce your weight and your risk of such conditions as heart disease, cancer, and stroke.

By replacing foods high in fat with complex carbohydrates (that is, any carbohydrate other than sugar) and proteins, you can eat the same amount while consuming fewer calories, gaining less weight, and helping to preserve your vision.

Eat less meat that is high in saturated fat and cholesterol, which acts to raise your cholesterol and clog arteries with the buildup of hardened plaque, also known as atherosclerosis. Meat also contains large amounts of iron, which oxidizes cholesterol into a form that is more easily deposited in the blood vessels throughout your body, further increasing plaque buildup. The blood supply to your eyes, which is critical in providing your vision, is adversely affected by plaque buildup. The result is clogged arteries and reduced blood flow. Last but not least, meat is low in antioxidants needed to preserve your vision and your general health.

If you must eat meat, eat more fish and poultry, which generally have lower fat content than beef, pork, or veal. Fish is preferable to poultry because it contains a type of fat called omega-3, which has been shown to reduce your risk of heart disease. If you do choose poultry, choose small portions of roasted or grilled skinless chicken or turkey breast. If you cannot give up beef or pork, choose the leanest cuts (like loin) and trim it of all visible fat before cooking.

Cut way down on processed foods such as crackers and potato chips, which are also rich in fat, particularly saturated fat and fatty acids, and can raise your blood cholesterol level in a fashion similar to meat. If you choose to eat these types of foods, look for those that are fat-free, or made without hydrogenated or partially hydrogenated oils, and eat them in moderation. Filling up on these types of snack foods leaves less room for the nutrient and antioxidant-rich foods essential for eye health.

Choose nonfat dairy products rather than their regular or low-fat counterparts. Half the calories in whole milk are fat.

Reduced-fat milk, which is often labeled "2 percent," actually has 38 percent of its calories as fat. Fat-free or skim milk is the only milk that is truly low in fat, and even though it is labeled fat-free, 2.5 percent of its calories is fat. So, if you drink a cup of whole milk, you get 8 grams of fat; you get 5 grams with the so-called 2-percent milk, but only .5 gram with fat-free milk. Most dairy products come in fat-free forms: yogurt, sour cream, cheese, and egg substitutes. You can use real eggs if you use just the whites. In fact, white omelets are quite popular at trendy restaurants these days.

Whenever possible, avoid oil, margarine, high-fat salad dressings, and high-fat dairy products such as butter, ice cream, and regular cheese. Oil is essentially liquid fat. When you need to use oil, select vegetable oils that are liquid at room temperature, since they have less saturated fat, and saturated fat raises your blood cholesterol level. Remember, your goal is clean arteries. Keeping your cholesterol down reduces the buildup of plaque in your arteries and also your chance of developing macular degeneration.

Be wary of food labeled "fat-free" until you check the serving size! Many manufacturers reduce the serving size in order to qualify the product as fat-free. The law currently states that any food containing less than .5 gram of fat per serving may be labeled fat-free. The reality is that the food may contain more fat than you are led to believe. And remember that "fat-free" does not mean "calorie-free"! Fat-free products can still be high in calories, and can result in weight gain and poor health when eaten in excess.

Avoid foods with more than 3 grams of fat per serving.

Join Leonardo, Paul, and Leo: Consider Vegetarianism

In general, fruits, vegetables, grains, and beans contain very little fat, and are preferred over animal products, processed foods, and oils. The only vegetarian products you will need to limit are oils, avocados, olives, nuts, and seeds, because of their high fat content relative to most vegetables. By adopting a vegetarian diet, you would join some celebrated company, including Leonardo da Vinci, George Bernard Shaw, Leo Tolstoy, and Paul McCartney and George Harrison.

A vegetarian diet can be highly nutritious and tasty, and can meet all of your nutritional needs. If you're not sure about adopting a vegetarian diet permanently, try adding several vegetarian meals each week to your diet, adding more as you realize how much you enjoy them! One of the benefits of a vegetarian diet is that because you are not filling up on red meats or poultry, you can enjoy more of the foods high in the antioxidants so important for preserving eye health.

When planning a vegetarian diet, be sure it's also low in fat. French-fried potatoes, for instance, qualify as a vegetarian food, but certainly are not a healthful choice. Plan your diet based on whole grains such as pasta and brown rice and whole wheat breads, accompanied by a wide variety of the highly nutritious fruits and vegetables recommended here. For protein, add nonfat dairy products, tofu and other soy products, and cooked dried beans, peas, and lentils.

SOME LOW-FAT SUBSTITUTIONS FOR HIGH-FAT FOODS

Foods rich in fat	Healthy low-fat substitute
Milk	Skim milk (can be enriched with a nonfat, cholesterol-free coffee creamer).
Cream	In cooking, use skim milk or evaporated skim milk.
Shortening or oil in baking (i.e., cookies, bread)	Fruit purees such as apple-sauce, plain nonfat yogurt.
White flour	Whole wheat flour for bread and pastry.

Foods rich in fat	Healthy low-fat substitute
Oil for sautéing	Fat-free cooking spray, fat-free broth, vinegars.
Cream cheese	Yogurt cheese or fat-free cream cheese.
Sour cream	Plain nonfat yogurt or fat-free sour cream.
1 whole egg	2 egg whites or ¼ cup of nonfat, cholesterol-free egg substitute.
Egg yolk for white sauce	Add a little egg substitute.
½ cup margarine	⅓ cup canola oil.
Stick margarine	For taste, use fat-free liquid margarine (does not work well for cooking or sautéing). For cooking/sautéing, use canola oil.
1 oz. baking chocolate	3 tablespoons nonfat cocoa powder plus 1 tablespoon canola oil.
Ice cream	Frozen low-fat yogurt, fresh-fruit sorbets.

You do not have to count calories and fat grams to achieve this goal; just follow some of the simple guidelines and make the low-fat choices suggested in this chapter. A few additional points to keep in mind:

- Always choose baked, broiled, steamed, poached, or grilled foods instead of fried ones.
- Use fresh or minimally processed foods whenever possible. When you buy processed foods, be sure to choose a low-fat or fat-free variety.
- Try fat-free liquid margarine instead of stick margarine or butter.

- Use nonfat cooking spray instead of oil for baking, cooking, or sautéing.
- Use fat-free or low-fat salad dressings, or a splash of flavored vinegar, to dress a salad.
- Fill up on fresh fruits and vegetables, especially a salad before dinner. This will not only give you extra antioxidants, but will leave less room for overeating a high-fat entree!

STEP 3

ELIMINATE RISK FACTORS WITH A HEALTHFUL LIFESTYLE

15

Begin a Regular Exercise Program

The evidence presented so far leads to an inescapable conclusion: daily lifestyle choices have more impact on vision than the medical community has realized. The health of your heart is intimately related to your visual health. A strong cardiovascular system enhances the delivery of nutrients to the eye and helps in the removal of waste products. And the number-one way to cardiovascular health is through exercise!

Despite the growing awareness of the importance of exercise to keeping hearts healthy, few people have made the link between regular exercise and vision. Regular moderate exercise is the first part of your program. The popular admonition "no pain, no gain" implies that if you do not "exercise until you drop," you are not getting anything out of an exercise program. This is simply not true. Programs that advocate intense exercise, just like the short-lived inspirations that happen around New Year's Day or after a medical scare, are often hard to maintain and may actually do more harm than good.

The Goal of Exercise

The goal of an effective exercise program is to build lean body mass, burn fat, and maintain cardiovascular health. Studies have shown that the healthier your heart and the cleaner your blood vessels, the less likely you are to develop visual loss from macular degeneration.

When you exercise intensely, your body responds by burning carbohydrates for its fuel, since carbohydrates take less time to convert into the necessary glucose. More-moderate exercise, however, allows your body to burn fat for the fuel it needs. Moderate exercise has also been found to decrease appetite (and hence food intake) and improve resting metabolism. Your resting metabolism is the rate at which your body normally burns calories; obviously this has a profound effect on both weight and overall health. Intense exercise, on the other hand, tends to slow your metabolic rate because, as an adaptive response to the heavy demand, your body tries to conserve energy; it does this by slowing down your metabolism. Finally, moderate exercise is safer, easier on your joints, feels better, and can improve your mood, self-confidence, and sense of well-being.

Which type of exercise is better overall, aerobic exercise such as walking, or resistance training? Aerobic exercise is more important because it does the most for your vision and overall health. So, if nothing else, commit to an aerobic activity on a regular basis. However, for optimum health and strength, a combination of moderate aerobic exercise, such as daily walking, and moderate resistance training two to three times a week can provide the best long-term results.

Remember, before starting this or any other exercise program, you will want to check with your doctor to make sure it is safe for you. This is particularly important if you are taking any medications, or are being treated for any existing health problems.

Aerobic Exercise

It is not hard to see that the basis of your exercise program should be moderate exercise. That is not to say that you must avoid more intense exercise, but that your primary objective should be a gentle aerobic activity such as walking. How much, and how often? This depends on individual ability, age, and preferences. Aerobic exercise is performed at a level where the body is able to deliver enough oxygen to meet the demands of the muscles. Over time, it helps condition the heart and lungs by increasing the efficient use of oxygen. The main criterion for aerobic exercise, then, is that it be continuous (i.e., nonstop). You may wish to start with fifteen minutes of daily walking, at a comfortable pace that does not leave you gasping for air. If you are breathless, it probably means your pace is too intense. Try talking as you walk. At the right aerobic level, you should be able to say three or four words in a row comfortably. Another helpful action is to check your heart rate. Your goal is to maintain your heart rate, during exercise, at 65–75 percent of the maximum rate for your age, which is calculated by subtracting your age from the number 220. Here's an example.

- Target heart rate (moderate exercise) for a 20-year-old: 220 – 20 = 200 × .65 to 200 × .75 = 130–150 beats per minute.
- Target heart rate for a 70-year-old (moderate exercise): 220 – 70 = 150 × .65 to 150 × .75 = 98–113 beats per minute.

As your fitness improves, you can increase both the intensity and the duration of the exercise, as long as you continue to breathe comfortably and your heart rate stays within the proper range. Thirty minutes or more of moderate aerobic exercise daily is ideal. Brisk walking is best, and is one of the best forms of aerobic exercise. Other effective types of aerobic exercise that many people enjoy, but some of which may take a toll on your joints, include cross-country skiing, rope-jumping, jogging, running in place, bicycling, rowing, stair-climbing, and dancing.

Resistance Training

Resistance training is any type of exercise that uses muscles to push or pull against an object that provides resistance—weights, for instance, including machines that incorporate weights. Resistance training is typically regarded as anaerobic (i.e., not aerobic) in form.

The goal of resistance training is to strengthen the muscle groups in the chest, back, shoulders, biceps, triceps, forearms, front thigh, hamstrings, calves, and abdomen. By strengthening muscle and increasing your lean muscle mass, you will burn more calories even while resting. Muscle is more metabolically active than fat. Resistance training also improves blood circulation. While not as important as the aerobic exercise prescribed in the MD Four-Step Program, moderate resistance training can be a useful supplement to aerobic exercise. Building muscle strength can also reduce pain from arthritis, prevent osteoarthritis, and make joints and bones stronger.

Engaging in this activity does not require a gym or costly equipment: you can buy dumbbells and large rubber bands (exercise tubing) inexpensively from most sporting-goods stores. Depending on the equipment available to you, your goal should be to start slowly (fifteen minutes, two to three times per week), and work up to thirty minutes or more per session as your endurance grows. If you choose exercise tubing, it will usually come with an instruction manual to help you get started on a resistance training program. Unlike daily aerobic exercise, you should take one day off between resistance training sessions to allow your muscles time to recover.

A Resistance Training Program You Can Try

This is a simple program that will help you strengthen your muscles and bones; it can be done by men and women of any age. When you start a program, perform only one set of twelve to fifteen repetitions of each exercise. As your strength and endurance increase, begin doing two to three sets of each one. Younger people may reach this point in two to three weeks, but it may take twice that long if you are older and out of shape. You should do resistance training two or three times a week, with a day of rest between workouts. This is important for your muscles. Once you are able to do three sets of fifteen reps with ease, increase the weight and decrease the reps to twelve. Then gradually go back to fifteen.

This is a simple program you can do at home with light dumbbells or resistance tubing. Some of the exercises use your own body weight for resistance.

For Your Legs

Chair Squat. Stand with your feet apart (about shoulder width) in front of a chair. Move your body as if you were going to sit down, but as soon as your backside touches the chair, return to the standing position. Do this fifteen times.

Leg Raise. Sit on the floor with one leg extended in front of you and one leg bent, foot flat on the floor. Place a rolled-up towel under your extended leg. Keeping your leg straight, raise it off the floor and the towel and hold it for ten seconds, then return your leg to the floor and the towel. Repeat for 12 to 15 repetitions for each leg.

Standing Side Leg Raise. Stand in front of a counter and place both hands on it for balance. Keep your torso erect and slowly raise one leg to the side as far as you can. Hold it for two seconds and return to standing position. Repeat 15 times with each leg.

Calf Raise. Stand on a step if you can, otherwise on the floor. If you are on a step, place the ball of your foot on the step with your heel over the edge. Drop your heel so you feel a stretch in your calf. Slowly raise your heel as high as you can and return to the starting position. Repeat 15 times with each foot.

For Your Upper Body

One-Arm Dumbbell Row. Using a light dumbbell of 5 to 15 pounds, place your knee on the edge of a sofa or bed. Bend over at the hip so that your back is parallel to the floor. Support your body with the hand on the side of the sofa. Place your dumbbell in your other arm and extend it toward the floor. Then raise it to your waist while bending your elbow and keep it close to your body. Return to the starting position and then repeat 15 times. Do the same thing with the other arm.

Chest Press. Lying flat on your back on the floor, hold dumbbells extended at arm's length out from your body to either side. Bend your arms 90 degrees at the elbow. Keep them just off the floor, and then bring them slowly together just over your head. Your arms should be straight, but not locked, at the top of the movement. Return to the start with your elbows just off the floor. Keep your wrist straight during this exercise. Repeat 15 times.

Dumbbell Biceps Curl. Standing or seated with your arms at your sides, bend your elbows and lift weights up to the front of your body. Do not let elbows travel forward. Return to the start. Do 15 repetitions.

Overhead Press. Hold dumbbells at shoulder level, with your elbows bent. Extend them upward and bring them together over your head. Don't lock your arms. Slowly return to the starting position and repeat 15 times.

Triceps Kickback. Using a similar position to the One-Arm Dumbbell Row, lean over a bed or sofa and bring your elbow to your side and "kick back" your arm so that it is extended straight behind you. Return to the starting position by bending your elbow 90 degrees. Repeat this 15 times with each arm.

Low Back Exercise. Lie flat on the floor, facedown. Raise one leg off the floor while at the same time raising your opposite arm (i.e., raise the left leg while raising the right arm, and vice versa).

Abdominal Crunch. Lie on your back on the floor, with your knees bent and feet flat on the floor. Place your hands on your thighs. Keeping your lower back flat against the floor, roll your shoulders up and forward until you can touch your knees with your hands.

16

Cultivate a Healthy Lifestyle Without Tobacco or Alcohol

The effect of smoking on the retina is devastating. As discussed in the section on risk factors, the retina is especially vulnerable to oxidative stress. Tobacco smoking adds to this stress and hastens the degeneration of the macular pigment and the development of macular degeneration. If you smoke, your macular pigment is only half as dense as that of a nonsmoker.

According to the World Health Organization (WHO), smoking is the cause of more death and disease than any other single habit. We have all heard about the evil effects of cigarette smoking on our lungs and heart, but there has been little mention of its effects on vision.

1. Smoking depresses carotenoid concentrations in the blood, even after adjusting for differences in diet.
2. Smoking increases oxidative stress, reduces plasma antioxidant levels, and increases the risk of vascular disease.
3. The adverse effects of smoking on vision are cumulative and not reversible.
4. A direct relationship has been found among the incidence of macular degeneration, the number of years a

person has smoked, and the number of cigarettes smoked per day.

5. People who live with a smoker are at a slightly greater risk than people who do not smoke or do not live with a smoker.
6. Nonsmokers have over twice the macular pigment density of the smokers.
7. Low levels of macular pigment contribute to increased risk of developing MD for smokers.
8. Smokers also tend to eat more fat than nonsmokers, but it was mostly men who were compared in the study that showed this correlation. Light exposure in an environment rich in fatty acids makes the cells in the retina particularly prone to oxidative stress.

The best way to reduce your risk of visual loss from macular degeneration and cataracts is to stop smoking now.

Ways to Quit Smoking

There are almost as many quit-smoking programs as there are diet books, and new ones are constantly appearing. It is not easy to quit, especially if you have been smoking for many years. Smoking is an addiction that can be as hard to beat as heroin or other hard drugs. However, it can be done if you get help. Most health professionals agree that the best way to quit is to combine behavioral techniques with nicotine replacement therapy.

Call your local chapter of the American Cancer Society or the American Lung Association for their booklets, videos, and other helpful materials. They also sponsor affordable group programs in most cities to help smokers quit.

Ask your doctor to help, too. You can now get nicotine replacement patches and chewing gum without a doctor's prescription, but you still need a prescription for the nicotine inhaler. This device, shaped like a cigarette, is designed to compensate for the hand-to-mouth action of smoking that is a major part of the habit.

How Alcohol Helps or Hurts Us

Bottled sparkling water and designer coffee have replaced much of the social drinking of alcohol that used to take place in this country, but there are still many people who like their cocktail hour—or two or three.

Moderation is the key with alcohol, but most people are not sure how that translates into actual drinking. For instance, can we drink equal amounts of beer, wine, and hard liquor? Is a frozen margarita more or less potent than two bottles of beer or glasses of wine? Most people cannot really define "moderate" because few really measure their drinks.

As we age, we become less tolerant of the effects of alcohol, and we feel those effects sooner. People using prescription drugs may metabolize alcohol differently from others. The alcohol could negate the action of a medication, or the medication could cause us to feel the effects of the alcohol sooner.

1. We know that a drink or two a day is good for the cardiovascular system, but more than that will cause health—and social—problems.
2. Women should have no more than one drink of alcohol a day because they have smaller livers, and a smaller volume of blood, so alcohol affects them sooner.
3. Just as heavy alcohol consumption can contribute to liver failure, heart disease, and a number of other ailments, it can also contribute to the development of visual loss.
4. Alcoholics harm their vision because they become malnourished and destroy most of the nutrients their bodies need. Chronic drinkers do not eat balanced diets, and alcohol also corrupts the digestive enzymes.

5. It is your liver that converts beta-carotene to the vitamin A that is so important to your vision, and with too much alcohol, this metabolism is interrupted.
6. Alcohol can also cause problems in the short term by decreasing vision or causing double vision, dilated pupils, night blindness, nystagmus (eyes moving back and forth rapidly), or paralysis of accommodation (our eyes' ability to adapt to images near or far and bring them into focus).
7. Alcohol limits the ocular muscles' ability to move the eyes up and down or from left to right.
8. Heavy drinkers are more likely to develop head and neck cancer.

For anyone who cannot or should not drink alcohol for any reason, the hazards of drinking alcohol daily obviously outweigh any potential benefits. Clearly, the proven beneficial effects of moderate alcohol consumption cannot be used as justification for inappropriate alcohol consumption!

There are currently a number of studies that indicate that an occasional glass of red wine—from once a day to once a month—can reduce your risk of heart disease and hence visual loss from macular degeneration.

Is Wine an Antioxidant?

Recently, results from the National Health and Nutrition Examination Survey (NHANES-1) found that the consumption of a moderate amount of red wine reduces the risk of macular degeneration by up to 34 percent. A combination of beer and wine, or liquor and wine, was found somewhat beneficial, but less so than red wine.

Red wine is known to increase the "good" cholesterol in the blood (HDL or high-density lipids), and this is what helps to prevent cardiovascular disease and keep blood vessels clean. Wine also contains antioxidant phenolic compounds, which contribute to its beneficial effect. Although the optimal amount for daily consumption was not determined in the study, I believe that if you are going to drink alcohol, based on the theoretical benefits of red wine and our knowledge of its protective effect on cardiovascular disease, one glass of red wine a day is the best choice.

Despite this study, I still believe that alcohol does more harm than good in the long run. My advice is to join the movement away from alcohol. The following pages offer a few alternatives that will help you prevent MD.

New Ways to "Drink"

Drinking is an excellent way to increase your antioxidant level. Drinking fruit and vegetable juice, that is! Replace gin with red or purple grape juice and a few crushed ice cubes to make a cool, refreshing drink with antioxidants. You can get some of the same antioxidant benefits found in wine by drinking purple grape juice (choose a brand with no added sugar, fortified with vitamin C) and eating red or purple grapes instead of green grapes. Fruit and vegetable drinks are an excellent source of beta-carotene, vitamins, and other nutrients. They provide most of the benefits of the whole product in a condensed form, so you are getting more value for the ounce. For example, six ounces of carrot juice contain more beta-carotene than two and a half whole carrots.

Water is, of course, the most important fluid for your body, and you should try to drink several glasses a day. Coffee and tea are fine in moderation, but the decaffeinated varieties will be your best choice if you drink more than one or two cups a day. Since coffee is a drug, too, replace that double latte with drinks that are high in antioxidants.

Here are some guidelines for making tasty antioxidant drinks:

1. Use a blender for fruit drinks and a juicer for vegetables. Soft fruits such as bananas, apricots, and plums

will clog the juicing machine. Pears, when firm, can be juiced, however.

2. Avoid juices made from foods rich in oxalate, such as beets, spinach, and chard, if you are prone to kidney stones.
3. If you are diabetic, use fruit juices sparingly because they are high in sugars.
4. Stir all drinks thoroughly before consuming.
5. Make juices ahead and refrigerate them for a day, or carry them in a vacuum flask. Remember, the longer drinks are stored, the more nutrients they lose.
6. Add a few crushed ice cubes to the mixture for a cool and refreshing drink, or put the ice into the blender with the fruit.
7. Always drink juices slowly. Vegetable drinks, in particular, can be unsettling to the stomach if taken too quickly.
8. Do not mix fruits with vegetables, with the exception of apples. Apples may be combined with carrots, celery, or other vegetables.
9. Melons do not mix well with other fruits.
10. Don't be afraid to experiment! You will enjoy creating your own blends. You will find some recipe suggestions for drinks in Part Three.

STEP 4

PROTECT YOUR EYES FROM VISIBLE LIGHT

17

Choose the Right Sunglasses

When was the last time you saw Bob Dylan without his shades? And what about the Blues Brothers? Are those dark glasses part of their "uniform," or are they meant to hide their eyes? When Ray-Ban introduced its trendsetting G-15 green aviator-style lens in the early 1950s, they worried that the public would not accept sunglass lenses that masked their eyes. The G-15 was significantly darker than other sunglass lenses of that era. How things have changed! Today sunglasses almost totally mask our eyes. In fact, that is part of what makes them fashionable, not to mention more protective. The G-15 marked a turning point when sunglasses were no longer considered beach equipment. It was the beginning of a new image for sunglasses as a serious protective device.

Sunglasses are a multibillion-dollar business. There are enough sunglasses manufactured to allow us not only the style we like, but the protection we need. There are entire stores dedicated to the sale of sunglasses. Finding the right pair among all the hundreds of choices is not an easy task. Salespeople rarely have a clue about protection from the sun, except to repeat the manufacturers' claims—and most claim their glasses will protect you from 100 percent of UV light. But there are no labels on many glasses, especially the higher-priced ones.

I began testing lenses by attending trade shows to visit the manufacturers' booths. In the process, I bought more than 100 pairs of sunglasses that looked as if they would meet the criteria I was looking for. I also went to Wal-Mart and a local supermarket, and a few sports stores to get less expensive ones for testing. (See Appendix 2 for my test results.)

When you buy sunscreen, the sun protection factor (SPF) is printed clearly on the label. With sunglasses, the information is less helpful. The claim that a lens "blocks 100 percent of ultraviolet light" can lead to a false sense of security. Protection from visible light is equally important, and yet most labels contain very little information about this factor.

Manufacturers of sporting sunglasses tend to make the best-quality lenses, probably because no serious skier would buy sunglasses of such poor quality that he or she could not see well. However, even glasses that allow you to see on the slopes and discern shadows and other visual details may not be protecting your eyes properly.

How reliable are the stickers and claims you find on sunglasses? In a review of children's sunglasses in 1991, it was found that thirty-three out of forty inexpensive lenses transmitted more than the stated amount of ultraviolet light, and one pair that said it filtered out "up to 98 percent" of UV radiation in fact let in nearly 10 percent.

What You Need to Know

Before you buy sunglasses, you need to think about which light rays can penetrate the lens, any color and shape distortion, the lens coating(s), and how the fit of the glasses protects your eyes.

Sunglasses provide more benefits than we think. First, they help to keep our vision sharp. In bright sunlight the retina becomes saturated with light, and the resulting image is less sharp. It's as if the brightness control on a television set were turned up too high. By reducing the light entering our eyes, sunglasses produce a sharper image, with better contrast. By protecting our eyes from bright light, sunglasses also help us adapt to low-light conditions later in the day. Graded-density sunglasses, which are darker at the top of the lens and more lightly tinted toward the bottom, can help reduce glare from sources above the line of vision.

Remember that to provide the best possible protection for your vision at all times and in all conditions, you will need more than one pair of sunglasses. For activities that take place in very bright sunlight, with lots of glare, you should have very dark lenses that will not be safe to use when driving. Therefore, your choice of sunglasses depends on the activity for which you will wear them.

For optimum protection, we would need both 100 percent shelter from UV light, to prevent cataracts, and 100 percent shelter from visible light, to prevent macular degeneration. Unfortunately the resulting lenses would be solid black, and we would not be able to see anything. What we need is the best possible balance between protection and comfort.

Because it is not possible to protect yourself completely from visible light if you want to see, your goal is to selectively reduce the amount of the more dangerous visible rays. Sunglass manufacturers rarely provide enough information to assist you in this decision. To help you in selecting sunglasses, I have spent countless hours analyzing numerous sunglasses to determine which lenses provide the best protection.

Lens Darkness

To make sure your lenses provide the best protection, select the *darkest* pair that is comfortable on a sunny day, while still allowing you to see traffic lights while driving. Don't rely on the store sales representative for this part of your selection process. Try the glasses on and ask if you can go outside the store and see how they work in sunlight. You cannot tell much inside a store with artificial light.

Your goal is to get a pair of sunglasses that transmits *12 percent or less visible light.* Here's a rough way to estimate if a pair of nonmirror-coated sunglasses meets this standard: Stand one to two feet from a clear mirror in a brightly lit room and look at your eyes through your sunglasses with your hand over the frame top to shield your eyes from overhead light. If the lenses are dark enough, you will not be able to see your eyes. I have tested a number of the more common sunglasses sold, and the amount of light they transmit is listed in Appendix 2.

Although darker is better for protection, you need to be careful not to overdo it. If the lenses are too dark, you are likely to miss seeing something such as a step or a ledge, and you could fall and get hurt. I have found the optimal balance between protection (darkness) and comfort for most people around town in southern Florida is a lens that transmits between 10 and 12 percent of visible light.

As mentioned in chapter 5, to protect ourselves from macular degeneration, we need to protect our eyes from blue wavelengths as well. However, if all the blue light is completely blocked, we cannot distinguish certain colors. Lenses that transmit between 2 and 5 percent blue light are ideal; they are comfortable to wear with minimal color distortion while providing the protection we need.

Blue light has a greater propensity to scatter when it hits an object, particularly small objects such as particles in the atmosphere, which is why the sky looks blue. Scattered blue light is largely responsible for haze, and skiers are particularly susceptible to scattered blue light. The more blue light is blocked, the crisper the vision.

Although the desired amount of visible-light transmission for sunglasses is less than 12 percent, where there is minimal reflected light, for example on a golf course, you may not need as much protection if you reduce direct overhead exposure with a visor or a brimmed hat—that is, so long as you do not spend an inordinate amount of time in the sand traps or water hazards, and are not constantly driving balls directly into the sunlight. However, for conditions where there is a large amount of reflected light, such as in snow, darker lenses with a transmission of less than 12 percent are more appropriate. Less than 7 percent would be even better. Remember, though, that when sunglasses let in less than 7 percent of visible light, they are not recommended for driving because you won't be able to see traffic lights correctly.

When the United States Army researched the effects of light on their night sentries during World War II, it found that strong sunlight could adversely affect night vision. In one report, a sunny day at the beach without sunglasses meant people needed one and a half times more light to see at night. Bright sun, researchers theorized, reduced the retina's sensitivity. In another report, sunglasses that transmit no more than 12 percent of visible light were found to protect the retina against this loss of sensitivity, while those that transmitted 35 percent or less did not prevent the loss. Light sensitivity is important because lower sensitivity may increase your risk of an automobile accident at night.

Lens Color

Photographers use colored filters to change the appearance of their subjects. Sunglasses do the same thing. Our brains automatically compensate for moderate changes in light conditions and color, so that for most sunglasses objects appear as we expect to see them. For example, a white towel looks white to us indoors under artificial light and outside under sunlight. Yet the artificial lightbulbs have much more red and far fewer blue wavelengths than natural sunlight. The white towel should appear yellow indoors. You could prove this by taking a color photo without using correcting filters or film. The camera, lacking your brain, does not compensate.

Color makes a difference when you are selecting sunglasses. And, again, you will want to choose lenses that provide maximum protection from blue light while still being comfortable to wear.

Manufacturers color their lenses in three ways: The lens may be dipped into a vat of dye; the coloring may be built right into the glass or plastic; or a special coating may be applied to the surface of the lens. Many outlets make prescription sunglasses by dipping the lens into a dye, and they often charge you a high price to do it. Lenses that are dipped eventually fade and need to be recoated. Lenses in which the tint is built in or is achieved using special coatings are best, and will not fade over time.

Tinted fashion eyewear is not the same as sunglasses. Such lenses offer no protection, and you should not assume that your optician can simply tint your lenses for protection.

Black. Black lenses may be the most effective at blocking out all types of light, but they block most of your vision as well. What we consider black glasses, however, are usually a very dark gray, because they do let some light through.

Orange and amber. My colleagues and I thought one of the best ways to prevent MD would be to use orange or amber lenses. These colors block not only 100 percent of UV light but also 100 percent of blue light, and would let in most of the safer remaining visible light to enable the wearers to get around. I began recommending orange or amber lenses to my patients. Although some loved them, most soon returned, complaining that these lenses not only failed to block sufficient light for comfort, but also distorted colors (blues became black, whites looked orange, and so on). Testing these "blue-blocking" lenses myself, I found I could not tolerate them either—the color distortion was too great.

Brown or tan. Brown or tan lenses, which block most but not all of the more damaging short blue wavelengths, provide an ideal balance between protection and comfort. I have found that a good pair of brown or tan lenses affords over 95 percent of the protective qualities of "blue-blocking" lenses, without the discomfort and color distortion. My patients who disliked orange lenses were amazed at the clarity and lack of distortion provided by brown or tan lenses.

Gray or green. Gray and green lenses are also acceptable, but do not provide as much protection as brown or tan lenses. Gray lenses produce the least color distortion, because they allow for equal amounts of all light to get through, and are preferred by some people. A good pair of green lenses provides protection similar to that offered by gray ones.

Yellow. Yellow lenses are reported to enhance contrast, and are favored by hunters on cloudy days. They do not provide adequate protection on sunny days, however. Scientists are puzzled by skiers' claims that yellow goggles make the world seem brighter on a cloudy day, because yellow allows only 80 percent of the light to come through, so, in effect, the world should seem less bright. In photography a yellow filter enhances contours in the snow, because through the yellow filter, shadows appear blue.

Blue and purple. Never, never buy these colors for use as sunglasses. Blue and purple lenses, though popular in some fashion circles, afford little if any protection for your eyes. A blue lens does not block blue light. Other colors, such as pink, pale green, or turquoise, may be fashionable, but these are not protective lenses. Wear them indoors if you wish, or on a rainy day.

Polarization

When I began researching sunglass lenses, I thought polarized lenses were more of a gimmick than a true benefit to vision. I quickly realized how wrong I was! Polarized lenses function like a venetian blind for your eyes. Only rays at a certain angle are let in, and this reduces glare. (Remember the Inuit whalebone shades mentioned in chapter 5?)

Polarized lenses are most useful where light is reflected

off flat surfaces, such as water, so they are popular among boaters. They are also excellent for driving, although some people dislike the spotted patterns (actually stress patterns) that appear on rear and side windows of the car when viewed through polarized lenses.

Sometimes polarized lenses can be a disadvantage. For example, ice produces its own polarized glare, so if you are driving on an icy road while wearing polarized lenses, you will not be able to see the ice as well. Also, because some airplane windows are polarized, polarized lenses may impair a pilot's vision.

Lens Material

Glass. Sunglass lenses are available in plastic or glass. Glass is heavier, less prone to scratches, and has been around longer. In my tests, glass tended to have the highest optical quality, which means it provided the sharpest vision. However, glass lenses do not always offer the best UV protection, and breakage can be a problem. For this reason they should not be used in sports, where breakage could result in irreversible damage to your eyes.

Plastic. I prefer plastic lenses because they are safer. They are also lighter, stronger, and better at filtering UV light. The disadvantage is that they scratch easily. As production techniques improve, the quality of plastic lenses will also improve. Many plastic lenses have almost the clarity of their glass counterparts. They are most often made from the following materials:

- **CR39** is the most common material, and is shatter-resistant and adequate for most uses.
- **Polycarbonate** is a "hardened" plastic and almost impossible to break. (Most polycarbonate will stop a .22-caliber bullet fired from a range of ten feet without breaking; no other lens does this.) If you engage in sports in which there is a risk of injury to your eye, polycarbonate sunglasses are for you. If you have lost vision

in one eye, polycarbonate sunglasses are excellent protection for your remaining eye. Polycarbonate lenses are particularly susceptible to scratches, so a scratch-resistant coating should be applied. If you have only one pair of sunglasses, this is the best choice for you.

- **Acrylic** lenses are more economical, and offer 100 percent UV protection that cannot be removed. Most of the more reasonably priced sunglasses on the market have acrylic lenses.

The labels may not say what material the lens is made from. If you tap a metal key against the lens, you will hear a ting from a glass lens, while plastic makes a duller sound. However, it may not be wise to do this in a store, because you may be thrown out.

Photochromic, or Transitional, Lenses

Photochromic (automatically darkening) lenses offer protection that varies with temperature and degree of sunlight. They are available in both plastic and glass lenses. Glass photochromic lenses work better than plastic. Plastic ones require direct sunlight to darken, so they won't work in your car. Photochromic lenses are most effective in cold climates because the higher the temperature, the lower the degree of darkening and the longer it takes.

If you are in love with your photochromic lenses, and are looking for the ideal environment to take advantage of them, snow skiing is the best place! The weather is cold, allowing them to darken fully and quickly when you are in direct sunlight, and they lighten later in the day, when the setting sun throws shadows on the ski slopes. If you find they are losing their effectiveness, put them in the freezer overnight and they should work better.

Gradient Lenses

Gradient lenses vary in degree of darkness from top to bottom. The most common are darker on top and lighter on the bottom. This reduces direct sunlight, allowing more light in along the "horizon" or the direction you are looking. Others are darker on the top and bottom of the lens, and lighter in the middle. Many of these are designed for use in snow, similar to the whalebone Eskimo device, and are ideal for any environment where there is considerable direct and reflected light, such as water, sand, or concrete.

Lens Shape

Sunglass lenses come in two shapes, flat and curved. Curved lenses are the most common. Except for frames with very small lenses, which are not ideal for protection, curved lenses provide clearer vision and the best protection.

Lens Coatings

All types of lenses can have coatings applied to increase their effectiveness, but not all lenses need them. Most mirrored coating—a thin metallic paint—has little effect on the amount of light transmitted through the lens, and is primarily cosmetic. Keep in mind that this coating has nothing to do with ultraviolet protection. In very bright environments, such as in the snow or on the water, mirrored coatings are reported to reduce glare.

Antireflective coatings can also reduce glare and are becoming more common. They are particularly effective when applied to the back of the sunglass lens. However, an antireflective coating makes it harder to clean your lenses, and you may want to avoid it if you wear your sunglasses for sports.

A scratch-resistant coating is a must for plastic (CR39, polycarbonate, acrylic) lenses, which tend to scratch easily. You should have both antiscratch and antireflective coatings on all plastic lenses that are not used for sports.

UV protection can also be added as a coating by dipping the lenses in a vat of hot PABA (para-aminobenzoic acid), the same substance found in sunscreens.

Frame and Lens Size

In sunglasses, one size does not fit all. The best way to see if a frame is suited for you is to try it on. Turn your head from side to side, and up and down. A pair of sunglasses that fits you well will not let in a great deal of stray light from any angle. If you can't try the sunglasses on outside the store, try to look for a spotlight or bare lightbulb, an "artificial sun," to test the frames and determine the degree of protection.

Frame size and the distance of the lens from your eye are important in controlling the amount of light that actually reaches your eye. By increasing the distance of a lens from your eye by only one-quarter inch, the light exposure can increase ten to twenty times.

The lenses should fit close to your eyes and preferably be large. I have found that even frames with smaller lenses can provide as much protection as larger frames, if they fit more closely to your face. Make sure the frame does not hit your eyebrows or your cheeks, as this will cause irritation after a while. Wraparound lenses provide excellent protection. If fashion rules and large lenses are out, wearing a cap or hat to shade your eyes can make up the difference.

I did not do any formal testing of the frames. In general, the cheaper sunglasses tended to fall apart just by putting them into and taking them out of the box I used to carry them around in. The more expensive frames did not have this problem. Nylon or thick plastic frames tend to hold up better than wire frames, and thick temples help to reduce reflected light. Hinged frames help prevent the glasses from breaking. If you are using them for sports, the weight of the frame may be important. Metal frames and wraparound frames tend to be the lightest.

Clip-on Lenses

Clip-on lenses are popular with people who wear corrective lenses all the time. These allow you to wear regular eyeglasses everywhere. When you go indoors or a cloud appears overhead, you simply flip the lenses up or snap them off.

Before you buy, consider the type of eyeglass lenses you use. Even when used with care, clip-on lenses will scratch most plastic lenses, and this is their greatest disadvantage. For this reason, glass lenses are a better combination with clip-ons. However, glass lenses are heavier and, again, put you at risk should they break.

Also, not all clip-on lenses were created equally. A study by researchers from Harvard Medical School showed that of nine clip-on lenses costing under five dollars, those made by Foster Grant performed best. Two-thirds of the clip-ons studied provided almost complete absorption of UV light, but one-third were inadequate, with transmission of up to 25 percent of some wavelengths.

Optical Quality

One way to test optical quality is to take the Amsler grid in chapter 2 to the store with you. After you have selected a pair of sunglasses, hold them six inches from one eye. Close the other eye, then hold the Amsler grid at arm's length from you. Make sure it is flat and well illuminated. Now move the sunglass lens around while looking at the dot in the center of the Amsler grid. Look through the center and the edges of the lens. If you do not have an Amsler grid, look at a straight vertical line (a doorway or telephone pole). With a good pair of sunglasses, the lines on the grid will remain straight, even around the edges of the lens. With a poor-quality lens, the lines will bend, curve, sway, move, and appear distorted.

Testing optical quality is the most challenging part of evaluating sunglass lenses. Overall, optical quality tends to be highest with glass lenses, although many name-brand companies offer high-quality plastic lenses.

Cheaper lenses tend not to be as well made. They are sold from large open display cases and get scratched as people try them on, whereas the more expensive lenses are typically locked up in a glass display case. Cheaper lenses are also not transported as carefully as their more expensive counterparts, which are packaged individually in their own boxes.

Cost

Sunglasses have a way of getting misplaced, and many people don't want to spend hundreds of dollars for them—especially if they need more than one type. Unfortunately, knowing what you are getting when you buy inexpensive sunglasses is difficult. In supermarkets and bargain stores, the sunglasses are on racks, and they are generically labeled. Unlike the high-end name brands, where each frame and lens type has a specific name, so that you know exactly what you are getting, inexpensive sunglasses do not.

The main reasons to spend a lot of money for sunglasses are to get better protection, good frames, and excellent optical quality. Some more-expensive brands give you this, as well as a more durable frame and optical quality. However, some of the least expensive sunglasses provide excellent protection, while some of the more costly ones offer less. Protection also varies within brands and even from one pair to another.

If you want protection more than style, there are inexpensive sunglasses that can meet your needs, and I have listed these in Appendix 2.

Prescription Sunglasses

In Appendix 3 you'll find detailed information if you need prescription sunglasses. Most people with contact lenses can buy regular sunglasses. But before you order prescription sunglasses you need to be sure the lens will offer you the protection you need while correcting your myopia or hyperopia. If you are nearsighted, the center of the lens will be thinner than the edges. As a result, the center you will be looking through will be slightly lighter in color than the edges. If you are farsighted, the opposite will be true; the lens will be darker in the center.

Knowing What the Labels Mean

Most manufacturers test their sunglasses using certain universal standards for visible light transmission and UV protection. If you are fortunate, the results will be present on a label. While the information is not sufficient to select a pair of sunglasses that meet the criteria of the MD Four-Step Program, it can be helpful. There are two widely used standards: American National Standards Institute (ANSI) in the United States and CE in the European Economic Community, and here is how to put this information to work for you.

In this country, meeting the ANSI standards is voluntary by the manufacturer. As a result, these standards can be misleading. A lens meets ANSI standards for UV blocking if it blocks as little as 60 percent of UVA light. The level of UVB blocking depends on the lenses' use. To meet the criteria of the MD Four-Step Program, the sunglass label must say the lenses *exceed* ANSI standards by blocking 100 percent of UV light. The American Academy of Ophthalmology recommends that we protect our eyes from all ultraviolet rays. Here is a look at the standards in this country and Europe:

ANSI STANDARDS

	% Transmission Visible Light	% Transmission UVA	% Transmission UVB
Cosmetic	100–40%	no greater than visible light transmission	no greater than ⅛ visible light transmission
General purpose	40–8%	no greater than visible light transmission	no greater than ⅛ visible light transmission
Special purpose	8–3%	no greater than ½ visible light transmission	no greater than 1%

Cosmetic and general-purpose lenses must also allow in 8 percent of red light, and 6 percent of yellow and green to ensure that drivers can see traffic signals. Color distortion is controlled to assure recognition of the signal. Special purpose lenses do not have to meet these requirements, and are not recommended for driving.

CE (EUROPEAN) STANDARDS

Number	% Transmission of visible light	Recommended use
0	100–80%	cosmetic
1	80–43%	cosmetic
2	43–18%	light-tint sunglasses
3	18–8%	regular sunglasses
4	8–3%	special-purpose, dark sunglasses (not for driving)

UVA transmission must be equal to or less than visible light transmission. UVB transmission must be equal to or less than ⅛ the visible light transmission.

Sunglasses that meet the ANSI *special purpose* standard or CE *level 4*, and state that they block 100 percent of UV light provide excellent protection. Any lens that meets these criteria will have a visible light transmission of 3 to 8 percent, which is well below my 12-percent target. Although these standards do not provide any information about the amount of blue light transmission, as long as the lens is brown, gray, or amber, you can count on it to provide excellent blue protection as well. Lenses that meet these criteria are great for skiing, snowy environments, and the beach. Unfortunately, they are below the recommended amount of light transmission for driving and are too dark for most people's comfort.

For driving, and for those who, like me, prefer lenses with 10 to 12 percent visible light transmission, the ANSI and CE standards are not as helpful. They can narrow down the field, but will not provide you with a definitive answer to whether or not they meet my standards for protection. The European *CE level 3* is a lot closer to what you should be looking for (visible light transmission of 8 to 18 percent) than the U.S. *ANSI general-purpose level* (visible light transmission of 8 to 40 percent). Remember, they must also block 100 percent of UV light. So if you prefer the 10-to-12-percent range, check the label. If it says *CE3* or *ANSI general purpose*, and blocks 100 percent of UV light, you are in the right range.

In the future, we can hope that manufacturers will give us more information on the visible and blue light transmission of the sunglasses we buy, so that it is easier to make sure we are getting the protection we need.

A Checklist for Buying Sunglasses

You've had to absorb a great deal of information in this chapter, and you probably should read it a few times to be sure you understand it all before you go and buy sunglasses. Here is a checklist with a review of what you need to know when you buy sunglasses, so that you are protecting your eyes not only from UV light, but also from visible light, and the risk of macular degeneration.

1. **UV protection.** Always get 100 percent UV protection. A tag that says "meets ANSI standards" is not good enough.
2. **Visible light transmission.** Buy the darkest sunglasses you can that will allow you to comfortably perform the activity you are planning. For regular wear, they should transmit no more than 12 percent of visible light *(ANSI special purpose* or *general purpose, CE level 3* or *4)* and between 2 and 5 percent of blue light. For driving, they should transmit between 7 and 12 percent of visible light *(ANSI general purpose, CE level 3)* so you can see the traffic signals.
3. **Color.** Brown or tan lenses offer the best balance between comfort and protection; gray or green is the

next best choice. Gray lenses are good for photography and painting, as they produce the least color distortion.

4. **Polarization.** This is preferred for everything except skiing, driving in icy climates, or flying in a plane with polarized windows.
5. **Lens material.** Polycarbonate is best overall, and for sports. Glass transmits a clearer image and scratches less easily, but is heavier and can injure the eye if it breaks. Glass is better suited for driving, traveling, sightseeing, and shopping. It is also better if you are a photographer or an artist.
6. **Photochromic (transitional).** These are not ideal for protection, and work best in cold climates. Glass photochromic lenses are best for driving. Plastic lenses do not darken except when exposed to direct sunlight, and so are not good for driving.
7. **Coatings.** All plastic (CR39, acrylic) and polycarbonate lenses should have scratch-resistant coatings. Mirror coating is good when sunglasses are for sports with a lot of glare, such as skiing or fishing. Antireflective coatings are good for driving or walking, but not for sports.
8. **Frames.** Bigger is better, but only if they fit closely to your eyes. Wraparound frames offer excellent protection.
9. **Clip-ons.** These will scratch plastic corrective lenses, and are best used in combination with glass lenses.
10. **Optical quality and distortion.** Check for distortion with an Amsler grid or by looking at a vertical pole to make sure there is no curve in the line.
11. **Price.** This has little to do with sun protection. Pay more only for better optical quality and more durable frames.

And Don't Forget Your Hat

A visor or baseball cap—worn with the bill in the front—will help to protect your eyes and reduce the amount of light that gets in around the frame. I am an avid believer in visors, and wear one anytime I go out into strong sunlight for any more than the length of time it takes me to walk from my car to a store or building. If you are protected by the shade of a brimmed hat, you can eliminate up to half the sunlight that would otherwise reach your eyes.

Does It Really Matter?

Georgia O'Keeffe, an artist who is best known for the wonderful images she painted of the New Mexico desert she loved, with its intense sunlight—and reflected light from the sand—developed macular degeneration. O'Keeffe refused to wear sunglasses because they distorted the color, such an important part of her work. Unfortunately, when she began to lose her vision, she followed an unproven eye exercise—fluttering her eyelids while looking into the sun—that probably hastened the development of her macular degeneration. Although she lived to be ninety-eight, O'Keeffe could not paint as well in the last decades of her life because of her macular degeneration, and this was the cause of a great deal of frustration. She also became paranoid, accusing others of stealing things from her because she could not see where she put them. Refusing to admit defeat, she stoically continued to paint, but with less detail, and with the help of assistants. However, few of O'Keeffe's late paintings have been shown. She eventually turned from painting to making pottery.

I don't know much about O'Keeffe's lifestyle, but I do believe that had she followed my MD Four-Step Program of antioxidants, low-fat diet, exercise, and protective lenses, she might have painted many more of her wonderful paintings and enriched all of us.

It's never too late, or too soon, to start my program. Don't let macular degeneration steal your sight. Start now, because the sooner you begin, the less likely you are to lose your vision to this devastating condition. I wish every one of you a long, healthy life, with excellent vision.

PART III

RECIPES TO PREVENT MACULAR DEGENERATION

Now it is time to put learning into practice! These recipes were created for you with the help of executive chefs recognized for their innovative health-conscious cuisine. Wherever possible, make the recipes with fresh vegetables, herbs, and other ingredients. Frozen ingredients should be your second choice, and canned goods should be the final option. Everyday items, such as salsa, are acceptable when premixed, but first check the label to make sure the item is low in calories and fat, particularly saturated fat.

As you become more familiar with a healthy diet, you can begin to experiment. Find ways to make your favorite recipes in a more healthful manner. For example, substitute ingredients that are lower in fat, such as skim milk for whole milk or cream, and fat-free cheese for its fatty counterpart. Add vegetables and fruits that increase your antioxidant intake, such as fresh spinach in a sandwich instead of iceberg lettuce. Improve the nutritional content of recipes such as stir-fried vegetables by including more of the vegetables that are high in antioxidants.

By exploring the recipe section and looking at the nutritional content of different items, you will get a better idea of ways to meet your nutritional goals. And once you are familiar with preparing food in a nutritious manner, it will be easier for you to create your own recipes, choose from among others, and order meals in a restaurant. Whatever you do, have fun and enjoy eating a healthy diet. Your eyes will thank you for it.

Nutritional Analysis

Nutritional analysis of the recipes was performed by Ginger Patterson, Ph.D., R.D., L.D., using "Nutritionist Five," a computer software program by First Data Bank, Inc., a subsidiary of Hearst Corporation, San Bruno, California. For each recipe, Dr. Patterson determined a value for calories, fat grams, percentage of calories from fat, beta-carotene, vitamin C, viatmin E, zinc, selenium, and manganese. The value for beta-carotene was determined using the retinal equivalent value reported by the program, then multiplying by 10 to convert it to IU. For vegetable drinks, it was assumed that half of the nutritional content would be lost in fiber that is discarded. Vitamin E is listed in IU, converted from ATE (1 ATE = 1 mg = 1.5 IU).

To determine lutein and zeaxanthin content, Dr. Patterson performed a manual calculation from values reported by Ann Reed Mangels in the *Journal of the American Dietetic Association.* At the time of publication, not all vegetables and fruits had been officially analyzed for lutein and zeaxanthin, so the value shown may be artificially low, and should be viewed as a relative value rather than an exact one.

RECIPE CONTENTS

Fruit Drinks

These are best prepared in a blender.

APRICOT DIVINE

RECIPE BY ERIC TRUGLAS

Rich in beta-carotene and vitamin C, this drink can be served for breakfast or lunch, or as a snack. The choice of apricots is not arbitrary, as they are among the best sources of beta-carotene.

8 dried apricots
1 Granny Smith apple
½ papaya, seeded (if not available, substitute mango)
3 ice cubes
1 tablespoon honey (optional—add to sweeten)

Soak apricots for 3 hours in 2 cups of water.
Peel apple and papaya.
Combine apricots with apple and papaya in blender.
Blend all ingredients on medium speed until smooth.
Add ice cubes, and blend for an additional minute.
Taste. If not sweet enough, add honey to sweeten.

MAKES 2 SERVINGS.

Serving size ¾ cup; Calories 186; Grams fat 0.481; % of calories fat 2%; Beta-carotene 2,586 IU; Lutein and zeaxanthin 0 mcg; Vitamin C 51 mg; Vitamin E 0 IU; Zinc 0.344 mg; Selenium 1 mcg; Manganese 0.145 mg

SWEETIE SMOOTHIE

RECIPE BY ERIC TRUGLAS

An excellent breakfast or snack drink, rich in beta-carotene. It goes well with bread or a muffin for breakfast.

1 large peach
1 banana
1 papaya (if not available, use mango)
1 orange
1 tablespoon honey
1 pint blueberries
6 ice cubes

Peel fruit, remove seeds, then dice.

Blend all ingredients together for 1 minute, then serve chilled.

MAKES 4 SERVINGS.

Serving size 1 cup; Calories 234; Grams fat 0.574; % of calories fat 4; Beta-carotene 492 IU; Lutein and zeaxanthin 0 mcg; Vitamin C 74 mg; Vitamin E 5.5 IU; Zinc 0.2 mg; Selenium 2 mcg; Manganese 0.279 mg

HAWAIIAN SMOOTHIE

RECIPE BY ERIC TRUGLAS

A good source of beta-carotene, excellent for snacks or breakfast.

1 cup pineapple, diced
1 papaya, peeled, diced (if not available, use mango)
1 mango, peeled, diced (if not available, use cantaloupe)
6 ice cubes

Blend everything together at medium speed for 1½ minutes.

Serve chilled.

MAKES 4 SERVINGS.

Serving size ½ cup; Calories 80; Grams fat 0.405; % of calories fat 5; Beta-carotene 2,216 IU; Lutein and zeaxanthin 0 mcg; Vitamin C 63.5; Vitamin E 4.2 IU; Zinc 0.101 mg; Selenium 1 mcg; Manganese 0.662 mg

Vegetable Drinks

Using the right vegetables makes these drinks excellent sources of antioxidants. They are good as snacks, or in combination with lunch. Milder-tasting juices made from carrots, celery, and apple juice are ideal to start learning about juices. Stronger vegetables, such as spinach and beets, are high in nutrients, but are best when consumed in small quantities in combination with the milder-tasting vegetables.

PLAIN CARROT JUICE

RECIPE BY ALEXANDER M. EATON

Carrot juice is sweet, and is great alone, without any other vegetables. An excellent source of beta-carotene, one glass a day provides all you need to fulfill the requirements of the MD Four-Step Program to preserve your vision.

3 carrots

Remove green leaves from carrots along with the very top of the carrot into which the green stems insert. Wash the carrots until clean, and insert in juicer.

MAKES 1 SERVING.

Serving size ¾ cup; Calories 64; Grams fat .284; % of calories fat 4; Beta-carotene 42,120 IU; Lutein and zeaxanthin 0 mcg; Vitamin C 14 mg; Vitamin E 2.0 IU; Zinc 0.3 mg; Selenium 3 mcg; Manganese 0.213 mg

CARROT TOP

RECIPE BY ALEXANDER M. EATON

My favorite vegetable drink. It is an excellent source of beta-carotene, and is very refreshing. It is good on a hot day, or following exercise.

3 carrots
2 Rome apples

Remove green leaves from carrots, along with the very top of the carrot into which the green stems insert. Wash the carrot tops until clean.

Rinse apples to remove chemicals, then slice and remove seeds and stalk.

Insert apples and carrot greens in juicer.

MAKES 2 SERVINGS.

Serving size 1 cup; Calories 72.9; Grams fat 0.39; % of calories fat 5; Beta-carotene 21,094 IU; Lutein and zeaxanthin 0 mcg; Vitamin C 11 mg; Vitamin E 1.65 IU; Zinc 0.177 mg; Selenium 2 mcg; Manganese 0.137 mg

POPEYE'S FAVORITE

RECIPE BY ALEXANDER M. EATON

A good source of beta-carotene, lutein and zeaxanthin.

3 carrots
½ cup of loosely packed spinach leaves

Remove green leaves from carrots, and wash until clean. Rinse spinach carefully. Make sure to remove sand. Do not remove stems. Insert in juicer.

MAKES 1 SERVING.

Serving size ¾ cup; Calories 66; Grams fat .310; % of calories fat 4; Beta-carotene 42,623 IU; Lutein and zeaxanthin 724 mcg; Vitamin C 17 mg; Vitamin E 2.4 IU; Zinc 0.35 mg; Selenium 3.5 mcg; Manganese 0.28 mg

VEGETABLE JUICE SPECIAL

RECIPE BY ALEXANDER M. EATON

Similar to V8 juice, but with twice the nutrients. It is rich in beta-carotene, lutein, and zeaxanthin.

1 stalk of celery
½ cucumber
4–5 medium-sized tomatoes (or 3 large tomatoes)
Small slice of lime (optional)

Remove the bitter outer leaves from the celery and use them to season a salad or soup. Then wash the stalk until clean. Wash cucumber, and slice in half. Remove the skin if the cucumber is waxed. Wash tomatoes, and slice. Remove stem. Add the slice of lime, if desired. Do not peel. Insert in juicer.

MAKES 2 SERVINGS.

Serving size 1 cup; Calories 38; Grams fat 0.55; % of calories fat 13; Beta-carotene 1,045 IU; Lutein and zeaxanthin 500 mcg; Vitamin C 32 mg; Vitamin E 1.0 IU; Zinc 0.226 mg; Selenium 1.5 mcg; Manganese 0.2 mg

PEPPER HEAVEN

RECIPE BY ALEXANDER M. EATON

Another of my favorites, rich in beta-carotene, lutein, and zeaxanthin.

5 carrots
½ green pepper

Remove green leaves from carrots, and wash the carrots until clean. Wash green pepper to remove chemicals, then slice and remove seeds and stalk. Insert in juicer.

MAKES 2 SERVINGS.

Serving size ¾ cup; Calories 58; Grams fat 0.26; % of calories fat 4; Beta-carotene 35,217 IU; Lutein and zeaxanthin 99 mcg; Vitamin C 27 mg; Vitamin E 1 IU; Zinc 0.27 mg; Selenium 3 mcg; Manganese 0.20 mg

GINGER DIVINE

RECIPE BY ALEXANDER M. EATON

A different twist, which is also very good, and an excellent source of beta-carotene.

5 carrots
½ apple
½-inch slice of fresh ginger

Remove green leaves from carrots, and wash until clean. Wash apple to remove chemicals, then slice, and remove seeds and stalk. Peel and remove skin, if waxed. Insert in juicer.

MAKES 2 SERVINGS.

Serving size ¾ cup; Calories 63; Grams fat 0.3; % of calories fat 4; Beta-carotene 35,108 IU; Lutein and zeaxanthin 0 mcg; Vitamin C

12.0 mg; Vitamin E 1.0 IU; Zinc 0.25 mg; Selenium 3 mcg; Manganese 0.18 mg

NIGHT VISION

RECIPE BY ALEXANDER M. EATON

An excellent source of beta-carotene, lutein, and zeaxanthin.

5 carrots
½ cup kale, mustard greens, or collard greens, loosely packed

Remove green leaves from carrots, and wash until clean. Rinse greens to remove chemicals.

Insert in juicer.

MAKES 2 SERVINGS.

Serving size ¾ cup; Calories 56; Grams fat 0.29; % of calories fat 5; Beta-carotene 35,453 IU; Lutein and zeaxanthin 1,835 mcg; Vitamin C 22 mg; Vitamin E 1.0 IU; Zinc 0.27 mg; Selenium 3 mcg; Manganese 0.18 mg

Appetizers

SWEET POTATO CHIPS

RECIPE BY ERIC TRUGLAS

An excellent source of beta-carotene, and a perfect snack.

4 sweet potatoes, washed and peeled and thinly sliced

Place potato slices on a baking pan. Oven-dry potato for 16 hours at 125–150° F. Should be crisp when done. If they are not crisp, try using thinner slices or cook longer.

MAKES 4 SERVINGS.

Serving size 1 potato's worth of chips; Calories 205; Grams fat 0.220; % of calories fat 1; Beta-carotene 43,631 IU; Lutein and zeaxanthin 0 mcg; Vitamin C 49 mg; Vitamin E less than 1 IU; Zinc 0.580 mg; Selenium 2 mcg; Manganese 1.120 mg

PAPAYA AND MOZZARELLA QUESADILLA

RECIPE BY ERIC TRUGLAS

Another of my favorites. An excellent source of beta-carotene. To make it more nutritious, try corn tortillas.

4 small fat-free flour tortillas
1 cup low-fat grated mozzarella cheese (do not use pregrated or sliced cheese)
3 papayas, peeled and seeded (if not available, use mangos)
½ ounce hot salsa
1 teaspoon fresh cilantro, chopped

Heat grill or grill pan on stove.

Preheat oven to 350° F.

Place tortillas on a counter. Spread with low-fat mozzarella and papaya. Cover each with salsa and fresh cilantro.

Place tortillas on grill to mark tortilla bottoms, or brown in a hot pan. Then fold in half and place on ovenproof plates and bake for 4 minutes.

Cool slightly, and cut quesadillas in quarters to serve.

MAKES 4 SERVINGS.

Serving size 1 tortilla; Calories 268; Grams fat 7.2; % of calories fat 24; Beta-carotene 1,091 IU; Lutein and zeaxanthin 0 mcg; Vitamin C 129 mg; Vitamin E 4 IU; Zinc 1.17 mg; Selenium 5 mcg; Manganese 0.188 mg

MIDDLE EASTERN TABBOULEH

RECIPE BY ERIC TRUGLAS

A good source of beta-carotene and vitamin C.

10 ounces precooked couscous
1 cup parsley, chopped
4 tomatoes, diced
½ cup scallions, chopped
½ cup mint, chopped
juice of 4 lemons
2 tablespoons extra virgin olive oil
3 each bell peppers, green, red, and yellow
black pepper

Mix all ingredients together.

Stir gently after 15 minutes.

Serve on a bed of lettuce or watercress with your favorite fat-free vinaigrette and black pepper to taste.

MAKES 8 SERVINGS.

Serving size 1 cup; Calories 121; Grams fat 3.9; % of calories fat 29; Beta-carotene 1,828 IU; Lutein and zeaxanthin 1,064 mcg; Vitamin C 135 mg; Vitamin E 2 IU; Zinc 0.46 mg; Selenium 1 mcg; Manganese 0.23 mg

EGGPLANT CAVIAR

RECIPE BY ERIC TRUGLAS

A good source of beta-carotene and vitamin C, this can be used as a dip for low-fat crackers, or served as a side dish. It can also be used as a sauce for fish.

4 eggplants
3 tomatoes
1 tablespoon olive oil

2 cloves garlic
2 shallots
½ onion
1 zucchini
1 yellow squash
white pepper
garlic salt or powder

Preheat oven to 350° F.

Cut eggplant in half, then place in a shallow pan and roast in oven for 10–20 minutes, depending on size of eggplant.

Remove inside of eggplant with a spoon and put in a mixing bowl.

Dice all vegetables and put in a skillet with olive oil. Sauté for about five minutes.

Flavor mixture with white pepper and add to eggplant in the mixing bowl.

Gently mix everything together and let cool. Add garlic salt or powder to taste.

MAKES 10 SERVINGS.

Serving size 1 cup; Calories 53; Grams fat 1.7; % of calories fat 29; Beta-carotene 665 IU; Lutein and zeaxanthin 318 mcg; Vitamin C 12 mg; Vitamin E less than 1 IU; Zinc 0.26 mg; Selenium 1 mcg; Manganese 0.228 mg

Soups

Soups can be served either as an appetizer or as a meal with a crisp green salad and fresh whole-grain bread. They are not only nutritious but easy to make. To save time, you can prepare a batch of your favorite soup and freeze some in small containers for future meals. Here is a simple, basic method for making soup.

Start with a prepared broth base, such as the Basic Vegetable Stock, or a nonfat, reduced-sodium canned broth, either vegetable or chicken.

Add fresh (or frozen) chopped vegetables—peppers, carrots, celery, or corn—finely chopped fresh herbs, and spinach or similar dark greens.

Add fresh (or canned) chopped tomatoes with their juice.

Add green peas, rinsed canned beans, or presoaked beans such as kidney, garbanzo, navy, or black beans.

As an option, add precooked pasta or brown rice just before serving.

Simmer for 20–30 minutes.

You now have an easy, nutritious meal, and you may have cleaned out your refrigerator at the same time!

If you like cream soups, use evaporated skim milk to reduce fat. Potatoes, boiled until tender, can be pureed in milk and used as a thickener. This could be the base for a delicious cream of broccoli soup that is high in beta-carotene. If you use milk, simmer at a moderate temperature to avoid scorching.

You can enhance the beta-carotene content of any soup recipe by adding carrots, chopped spinach, and fresh herbs; the lutein content can be boosted by adding sliced or chopped celery or spinach.

Homemade soups are easy, so don't be afraid to experiment. You may just find a new favorite.

TOMATO AND WATERCRESS SOUP WITH FRESH BASIL

RECIPE BY ERIC TRUGLAS

One of my favorites, good with salad and bread for lunch, this soup is an excellent source of beta-carotene and vitamin C.

2 heads garlic
2 teaspoons olive oil for garlic

1 onion, peeled and chopped
2 celery stalks, chopped
4 carrots, chopped
16 ounces watercress leaves
3 red peppers, chopped
8 ounces tomato ketchup
1 tablespoon olive oil
1 cup water
1 cup white wine
2 tablespoons chopped fresh basil
pinch of garlic salt
pinch of white pepper
chopped fresh basil for garnish

Preheat oven to 350° F.

Remove loose skin from garlic. Cut each head in half, crosswise, and place on baking sheet. Drizzle each half with 1 teaspoon olive oil. Roast for 20 minutes.

In a medium bowl, press garlic from each clove; combine with onion, celery, carrot, watercress, red pepper, and tomato ketchup.

In a soup kettle, heat olive oil over moderate heat. Add the vegetable mixture and cook 5 minutes.

Add water and wine. Bring to boil over high heat, then reduce heat and simmer 15 minutes, covered.

Put soup into blender (in batches if necessary), and puree.

Pour soup back into kettle. Add chopped basil, garlic salt, and pepper. Simmer over moderate heat 5 minutes.

Serve hot in soup bowls, with chopped basil sprinkled on top as garnish.

Makes 6 servings.

Serving size 1 cup; Calories 179; Grams fat 4.307; % of calories fat 22; Beta-carotene 23,049 IU; Lutein and zeaxanthin 476 mcg; Vitamin C 94 mg; Vitamin E 4 IU; Zinc 0.591 mg; Selenium 2 mcg; Manganese 0.8 mg

ROASTED TOMATO BISQUE

RECIPE BY TODD JOHNSON

8 vine-ripened tomatoes, cut in half
1 teaspoon garlic, minced
1 whole shallot, minced
4 sprigs fresh thyme, destemmed and chopped
¾ ounce fresh basil, thinly sliced
½ cup olive oil
2 whole Spanish onions, diced
½ cup flour
4 cups fat-free chicken broth
1 cup skim milk
¼ cup tomato paste
salt and pepper

Preheat oven to 250 degrees.

Place halved tomatoes on a baking sheet, flat side down.

In a small bowl, mix the garlic, shallot, thyme, and basil with ¼ cup olive oil.

Drizzle this mixture over the tomatoes, and bake for 2 hours.

While the tomatoes are baking, in a large pot sauté the chopped onions for 5 minutes in ¼ cup olive oil. Add the flour and stir in.

Add the chicken broth, skim milk, roasted tomatoes, and tomato paste.

Simmer soup for 20 minutes, then puree in a blender and add salt and pepper to taste.

MAKES 8 SERVINGS.

Serving size 1 cup; Calories 88; Grams fat 0.607; % of calories fat 6; Beta-carotene 2,281 IU; Lutein and zeaxanthin 95 mcg; Vitamin C 269 mg; Vitamin E 0.565 IU; Zinc 0.382 mg; Selenium 3 mcg; Manganese 0.275 mg

GAZPACHO

RECIPE BY ERIC TRUGLAS

Another of my favorites, and an excellent source of beta-carotene, lutein and zeaxanthin.

6 ounces cooked pumpkin meat (see instructions below; substitute frozen or canned if fresh is not available)
3 carrots
1 cucumber
1 red pepper
4 celery stalks
½ yellow onion
½ cup lime juice
2 tablespoons tomato paste
1 tablespoon olive oil
1 quart (32 ounces) low-sodium canned V8® juice
pepper and salt

To prepare the pumpkin:

Use a small pumpkin, the size of a cantaloupe.

Cut out a hole around the stem, then scoop out and discard the pumpkin seeds.

Bake the pumpkin at 375° F for 30–40 minutes, until it is tender and the meat of the pumpkin can easily be pierced with a fork. Alternatively, you can cook it in a microwave on a vegetable setting for 2–3 minutes until tender.

Cut the pumpkin in half. Scoop out the meat using a spoon.

To complete the dish:

Mince vegetables and place in a large bowl.

Add the rest of the ingredients, and mix. Put the mixture in a food processor and pulse on and off (in batches if necessary), until chunky consistency is achieved.

Season with pepper and salt. Chill well.

Serve cold.

MAKES 7 SERVINGS.

Serving size 1 cup; Calories 108; Grams fat 4.120; % of calories fat 34; Beta-carotene 15,276 IU; Lutein and zeaxanthin 1,185 mcg; Vitamin C 64 mg; Vitamin E 3 IU; Zinc 0.565 mg; Selenium 1 mcg; Manganese 0.319 mg

HARVEST VEGETABLE SOUP

RECIPE BY JOY PURCELL

A glorious array of fresh, healthy vegetables goes into the soup pot. Lentils or beans make this a very satisfying meal.

1 onion, peeled and medium diced
2 carrots, peeled and medium diced
1 leek, cut in half lengthwise, washed very well, diced
3 celery stalks, sliced in medium pieces
1 tablespoon olive oil
3 cloves garlic, crushed
1 zucchini, medium diced
1 summer squash, medium diced
1 cup corn kernels
1 cup peas
10 ounces spinach, chopped (frozen spinach may be substituted)
15 ounces canned tomatoes, no salt added
1 cup lentils or canned cannelloni beans
1 quart nonfat vegetable or chicken broth
3 tablespoons fresh basil, chopped fine
fresh ground pepper

In a large saucepan, sauté the onion, carrots, leek, and celery in the oil until aroma is given.

Add garlic next, cooking for a few minutes. Add all other vegetables and lentils or beans.

Add tomatoes and broth, cover and simmer until all vegetables are tender and lentils are done.

You may need to add more broth. The lentils do absorb some liquid. Adjust the liquid accordingly. There should be enough liquid so the vegetables have a little room to float.

When the soup is ready, garnish with fresh basil, add pepper to taste, and adjust your seasoning.

This recipe has no salt in it. For flavor enhancement, try adding a little fresh lemon juice, balsamic vinegar, or Tabasco sauce.

MAKES 8 SERVINGS.

Serving size 8 ounces; Calories 151; Grams fat 2.242; % of calories fat 13; Beta-carotene 6,906 IU; Lutein and zeaxanthin 5,100 mcg; Vitamin C 22 mg; Vitamin E 1.5 IU; Zinc 1.002 mg; Selenium 3 mcg; Manganese 0.710 mg

CREAM OF FRESH PEA SOUP

RECIPE BY JOY PURCELL

A beautiful pale green soup with a hint of springtime and a fresh light flavor. It is pureed using low-fat alternatives to the traditional heavy cream. High in lutein and zeaxanthin, the soup perfectly combines health, quality, and taste.

2 pounds fresh or frozen peas
2 cups nonfat vegetable or chicken broth
1 cup evaporated skim milk
salt, to taste
1 tablespoon fresh chives, chopped
1–2 tablespoons fresh mint, sliced very fine
1 red pepper, seeded and finely diced
1 yellow pepper, seeded and finely diced

In a microwave or steamer, cook the peas until they are bright green and just tender.

Blend the vegetables in a food processor or blender until they are smooth, adding a little broth so they will incorporate easily. You may burn out your blender if the mixture is too thick, so do it in two batches if necessary.

In a saucepan, heat the broth and add the fresh pea puree. Bring to a simmer, stirring often to keep from scorching.

When the soup is hot add evaporated skim milk to finish it off. Do not boil the milk or it will curdle.

Garnish with chives, mint, and peppers; serve in warmed bowls.

MAKES 6 SERVINGS.

Serving size 8 ounces; Calories 168; Grams fat 0.603; % of calories fat 3; Beta-carotene 1,788 IU; Lutein and zeaxanthin 2,722 mcg; Vitamin C 91 mg; Vitamin E less than 1 IU; Zinc 1.875 mg; Selenium 2 mcg; Manganese 0.690 mg

SPINACH AND MUSHROOM SOUP

RECIPE BY JOY PURCELL

This soup utilizes mushrooms, herbs, and tomatoes to make a flavorful broth. Spinach is added at the end for color, a touch of difference, and many nutrients. Easy to make, light and tasty, the soup is a must to try.

1 tablespoon olive oil
2 onions, peeled and chopped
3 leeks, washed and chopped
3 cloves garlic, crushed
2 pounds mushrooms, washed and chopped
2 teaspoons dried marjoram
1/4 teaspoon dried thyme
1/4 cup Madeira (or sherry, Marsala, or red wine)
3 tablespoons tomato paste
1 bay leaf
2 quarts nonfat vegetable broth
1 pound fresh spinach, washed well, stems removed, and sliced very fine

In a large saucepan, heat oil over medium heat, add onions, leeks, and garlic. Cover, and let the natural juices steam them for about 20 minutes. Browning may occur, so stir often to prevent scorching.

Stir in mushrooms and seasonings. Cook until the mushrooms give off liquid. Turn heat down and cook 5 minutes.

Add the Madeira. Simmer the mixture a few minutes to reduce the amount of alcohol.

Add tomato paste and bay leaf, then stir to blend.

Add broth and simmer for 45 minutes.

Strain soup through a strainer, pressing on the vegetables to extract all the liquid. Discard the vegetables.

Bring soup to a simmer and add the fresh spinach, then serve immediately.

Garnish with fresh sliced mushrooms if you like.

MAKES 6 SERVINGS.

Serving size 8 ounces; Calories 162; Grams fat 4.746; % of calories fat 26; Beta-carotene 5,338 IU; Lutein and zeaxanthin 8,580 mcg; Vitamin C 38 mg; Vitamin E less than 1 IU; Zinc 1.730 mg; Selenium 23 mcg; Manganese 1.212 mg

BASIC VEGETABLE STOCK

RECIPE BY JOY PURCELL

This stock is used as a base for vegetarian soups and sauces. The vegetables vary, so you can use any trimmings or leftovers. Good to have on hand, and it freezes well.

1 cup onions (you can use onion peels if you want a golden color)
1 cup leeks, carefully washed (save the trimmings for this purpose)
1 cup celery, use ends and leaves
3/4 cup cabbage (can impart a strong flavor)
1 cup carrots (use peelings, end pieces, etc.)

1 cup turnips, all parts
1 cup tomatoes, all parts
4–5 cloves garlic (use skins also)
1 gallon water (approximately)

Place all ingredients in a saucepan, add enough water to cover vegetables, and simmer slowly for 1–2 hours. Strain, then refrigerate until needed for a recipe. This stock can be frozen. Varying the ingredients will make a change in the flavor of the dish.

MAKES 16 SERVINGS.

Serving size 1 cup; Calories 4.25; Grams fat 0.028; % of calories fat 6; Beta-carotene 505 IU; Lutein and zeaxanthin 100 mcg; Vitamin C 1 mg; Vitamin E less than 1 IU; Zinc 0.025 mg; Selenium 0.25 mcg; Manganese 0.025 mg

Breads

ASSORTED FRUIT QUICK BREAD

RECIPE BY JOY PURCELL

Interesting flavor and nicely textured, this bread is excellent for toast, and makes an attractive gift. An easy bread to make.

½ cup fat-free liquid egg substitute
¼ cup granulated sugar
1 tablespoon nonfat liquid margarine
1 cup unbleached all-purpose flour
½ cup whole wheat flour
1½ teaspoon double-acting baking powder
¼ teaspoon cinnamon
¼ teaspoon ginger
1 teaspoon salt
10 ounces fruit bits mix (containing apricots, peaches, apples, and raisins)
1 cup warm water

Presoak the dried fruit in warm water for 30 minutes; drain and reserve water for later use.

Line a 9 × 5 × 3 bread pan with parchment paper and spray with nonstick cooking spray.

With an electric mixer, beat egg substitute and sugar until they are light and fluffy.

Sift flours, baking powder, cinnamon, ginger, and salt together.

Add flour mixture along with the nonfat liquid margarine to the eggs and sugar.

Add all the dried fruit, and fold in all ingredients gently until just blended (do not overwork the batter). If the bread batter is very stiff, add a little of the reserved water, about ¼ cup.

Pour into the prepared pan and bake in a preheated 350° F oven for 30–40 minutes. Cooking times vary among different ovens, so after the time is up, insert a toothpick into the bread. If the toothpick comes out clean, the bread is done; if not, bake a little longer.

Cool slightly in the pan, then remove the loaf to a rack to finish cooling.

MAKES 1 LOAF (APPROXIMATELY 16 SLICES).

Serving size 1 slice; Calories 102; Grams fat 0.238; % of calories fat 2; Beta-carotene 554 IU; Lutein and zeaxanthin 0 mcg; Vitamin C 0.650 mg; Vitamin E less than 1 IU; Zinc 0.322 mg; Selenium 0.001 mcg; Manganese 0.253 mg

SWEET POTATO MUFFINS

RECIPE BY JOY PURCELL

These muffins have a beautiful color, and a lovely aroma when cooking. You can substitute pumpkin for the sweet potato with very good results. A high source of beta-carotene, these muffins are a great way to start any day for nourishment and flavor.

1 cup unbleached all-purpose flour
½ cup whole wheat flour
½ cup firmly packed brown sugar
2 teaspoons double-acting baking powder
2 teaspoons cinnamon
½ teaspoon ginger
½ teaspoon ground cloves
1 teaspoon salt
1 cup cooked mashed sweet potato or pumpkin
½ cup skim milk
¼ cup nonfat egg substitute
1 tablespoon canola oil
¾ cup raisins (optional)

Preheat oven to 350° F.

Prepare muffin pans with nonstick cooking spray.

Combine flours, sugar, baking powder, cinnamon, ginger, cloves, and salt in a large bowl and mix well.

Make a well in the center of the mixture.

Combine sweet potato or pumpkin, skim milk, egg substitute, and canola oil in a separate bowl, making sure to mix thoroughly.

Spoon the sweet potato mixture into the well in the middle of the dry ingredients, and stir just until moistened. (Add the raisins also, if you are including them.)

Spoon batter into muffin pans, filling about ¾ full.

Bake for about 20 minutes. Check for doneness.

Remove muffins from pan immediately. Serve warm or at room temperature.

MAKES 12 SERVINGS.

Serving size 1 muffin; Calories 163; Grams fat 1.5; % of calories fat 8; Beta-carotene 4,774 IU; Lutein and zeaxanthin 0 mcg; Vitamin C 5.2 mg; Vitamin E less than 1 IU; Zinc 0.438 mg; Selenium 0.001 mcg; Manganese 0.521 mg

Salads and Dressings

SALADS AND FRESH HERBS

Salads are an excellent source of beta-carotene, lutein, and zeaxanthin, and you should eat two a day. Make them a part of every lunch and dinner you have, unless your doctor has instructed you not to eat salads. (If you are taking Coumadin, which is a blood thinner, check with your doctor before eating two salads a day. Also, certain gastrointestinal disorders limit raw vegetable intake.)

A simple salad of a half-ounce each of spinach and leaf lettuce, and one medium tomato, contains 1,774 IU of beta-carotene and 1,804 mcg of lutein and zeaxanthin. Add one carrot, and the beta-carotene content increases to 36,338 IU. It is as simple as this: Eat two such salads and you can meet your minimum dietary requirement of beta-carotene, lutein, and zeaxanthin for the day.

DRESSINGS

Because of the tremendous benefit of salads, you can be a little lenient with the calorie and fat content of dressings. The benefit of eating two salads a day far outweighs the downside of a few more calories and a little fat. For optimal benefit, however, fat-free dressings are best. Buy them at the supermarket, or make them yourself. To reduce the fat content of your dressing, reduce the amount of oil you use, or eliminate it altogether.

Use a variety of salad dressings to liven up the dish and take the monotony out of eating two a day. Here's an easy way to make the base for your own:

Make a mixture of 3 parts good balsamic (or white or red wine) vinegar to 1 part virgin olive oil. Add water to dilute, about half the amount of vinegar you started with. Add a dash of spices, such as dill and basil, and a squeeze of lemon (fresh spices are best, but dried ones will work as well). Add salt and pepper to taste, and a dash of garlic. A spoonful of Dijon mustard makes a great addition. A small spoonful of honey or sugar will reduce the sharp taste of the vinegar, and will balance the flavors. Mix together.

Now you can start creating your own dressings. Remember, the less oil you use, the less fat you take in and the better it is for you.

Serving Salads

To keep the amount of salad dressing at a minimum, gently toss the salad mix in a large bowl with a vinaigrette or other dressing of your choice, then serve the salad in a platter or in individual bowls. This uses less dressing than topping an individual salad.

Vinaigrettes make an excellent seasoning for fish, chicken, vegetables, rice, or pasta and can be served warm as well as cold.

HONEY-DIJON MUSTARD DRESSING

RECIPE BY ERIC TRUGLAS

¾ cup Dijon mustard
¼ cup fresh dill
¼ cup fresh basil
¼ cup white vinegar
½ cup honey
¼ cup canola or olive oil
1¼ cups water

Blend mustard, herbs, white vinegar, and honey in a blender or food processor.

With machine on high setting, slowly add oil in a thin stream, then add water.

The dressing should be about the consistency of mayonnaise. If it is too thick, add more water.

MAKES 3 CUPS.

Serving size 2 tablespoons; Calories 71; Grams fat 5.1; % of calories fat 64; Beta-carotene 27 IU; Lutein and zeaxanthin 6 mcg; Vitamin C less than 1 mg; Vitamin E 1 IU; Zinc 0.131 mg; Selenium 5 mcg; Manganese 0.038 mg

BALSAMIC VINAIGRETTE

RECIPE BY ERIC TRUGLAS

An excellent choice. This dressing can be refrigerated, as it stores well.

2 tablespoons Dijon mustard
1 tablespoon extra virgin olive oil
3 tablespoons balsamic vinegar
½ tablespoon each chopped thyme, oregano, and basil
1 shallot, chopped
salt and pepper

Whisk all ingredients together; taste; add salt and pepper to suit. Store covered in refrigerator.

MAKES ⅜ CUP.

Serving size 2 tablespoons; Calories 73; Grams fat 5.255; % of calories fat 64; Beta-carotene 21 IU; Lutein and zeaxanthin 0 mcg; Vitamin C less than 1 mg; Vitamin E less than 1 IU; Zinc 0.153 mg; Selenium 0 mcg; Manganese 0.006 mg

TROPICAL BLEND CREAMY DRESSING

RECIPE BY JOY PURCELL

A light, sweet-tart dressing that is creamy and tasty. Using alternatives to fats and oils, the dressing is made with pureed fruits and nonfat plain yogurt. The flavors go well with dark leafy salads and bitter greens.

½ cup fresh-squeezed orange juice
3 ounces ripe fresh mango, papaya, guava, or apricots, peeled, with seeds removed
⅓ cup white wine vinegar
½ teaspoon mace
¼ teaspoon white pepper
½ cup plain nonfat yogurt
½ small banana (optional, adds a wonderful subtle flavor)

Blend all ingredients in a blender or food processor until thoroughly smooth. Pour into a small bowl and chill for a few hours.

Serve over salad. Garnish your salad with mandarin orange segments for a different look.

This dressing should be used right away to ensure fresh quality.

MAKES 6 SERVINGS.

Serving size 2 ounces (4 tablespoons); Calories 40; Grams fat 0.173; % of calories fat 4; Beta-carotene 601 IU; Lutein and zeaxanthin 0 mcg; Vitamin C 15 mg; Vitamin E less than 1 IU; Zinc 0.219 mg; Selenium 5 mcg; Manganese 0.024 mg

TOMATO BASIL VINAIGRETTE DRESSING

RECIPE BY JOY PURCELL

We replaced the oil used in standard vinaigrette with fresh herbs and vegetables, transformed to make a light and flavorful alternative to the standard dressing. This dressing falls into all the categories for vitamin C, beta-carotene, and lutein and zeaxanthin, and it goes well with Boston, Bibb, or romaine lettuce. For an interesting zip, add a little fresh ginger.

3 teaspoons canola oil
2 cloves garlic, minced
½ small red onion, peeled and finely chopped
2 tablespoons tomato paste
3 ripe large tomatoes, peeled, seeded, and chopped
2 tablespoons fresh basil, finely chopped
3 teaspoons cilantro, finely chopped
1 teaspoon tarragon, finely chopped
¼ cup balsamic vinegar

In a medium sauté pan, heat the oil and add the garlic and onion. Cook until an aroma begins to rise.

Add the tomato paste and sauté briefly. Do not allow it to brown.

Add the tomatoes, and simmer until the mixture reduces by one-quarter. Reducing the liquid will concentrate the flavors.

Allow the tomato mixture to cool slightly, then puree in a blender until smooth.

Add fresh herbs and vinegar when completely cooled, and adjust seasoning.

MAKES ABOUT 1 CUP.

Serving size 2 ounces (4 tablespoons); Calories 85; Grams fat 3.801; % of calories fat 40; Beta-carotene 837 IU; Lutein and zeaxanthin 95 mcg; Vitamin C 23 mg; Vitamin E 2 IU; Zinc 0.212 mg; Selenium 1 mcg; Manganese 0.203 mg

TUNA SALAD WITH TROPICAL FRUIT

RECIPE BY ERIC TRUGLAS

An excellent source of beta-carotene, this is excellent on pita bread as a sandwich, or as a dip for snacks.

2 6½-ounce cans white tuna in water, drained
1 cup papaya, peeled, seeded, and diced
1 cup mango, peeled, seeded, and diced
1 cup celery, chopped
1 cup shredded carrots
¼ cup chopped green onions
¼ cup chopped red onion
¾ cup low-fat mayonnaise
1 teaspoon curry powder
1 bunch collard greens, washed and set aside

Combine tuna, papaya, mango, celery, carrots, chopped green onions, and red onion in a bowl.

Combine the mayonnaise and curry powder in a small bowl. Add to the tuna mixture and toss gently to mix.

Cover and chill. Spoon the salad into a serving dish lined with collard greens.

MAKES 8 SERVINGS.

Serving size ¾ cup; Calories 195; Grams fat 9.006; % of calories fat 41; Beta-carotene 9,259 IU; Lutein and zeaxanthin 541 mcg; Vitamin C 35 mg; Vitamin E 4 IU; Zinc 0.333 mg; Selenium 34 mcg; Manganese 0.063 mg

THAI CHICKEN SALAD

RECIPE BY ERIC TRUGLAS

Great with steamed rice. If you have a sweet tooth, this salad is for you. An excellent source of beta-carotene and vitamin C.

½ cup marmalade
½ cup lime juice
1 teaspoon chopped ginger
1 teaspoon ground nutmeg
1 dash Tabasco sauce
1 teaspoon olive oil
4 chicken breasts, diced
4 papayas, diced (if not available, use mango)
4 cooked carrots, diced
1 cup fresh chopped cilantro

In a small saucepan, melt marmalade over low heat, gradually blending in lime juice, ginger, nutmeg, and Tabasco sauce.

Heat olive oil in skillet and brown the chicken, then add papaya and carrots and blend with the marmalade mixture.

Cook over medium heat for 6 to 8 minutes.

Spoon on serving dish and sprinkle with fresh cilantro.

MAKES 4 SERVINGS.

Serving size 1½ cups; Calories 477; Grams fat 4.235; % of calories fat 8; Beta-carotene 17,149 IU; Lutein and zeaxanthin 0 mcg; Vitamin C 181 mg; Vitamin E 6 IU; Zinc 2.045 mg; Selenium 2 mcg; Manganese 0.567 mg

Vegetarian Entrees

All sautéed items should be prepared in nonstick pans to minimize the use of butter, oil, or other fatty products.

An excellent source of beta-carotene, lutein, and zeaxanthin, these vegetables are great by themselves, but at Bistro

41 we like to put a fresh piece of fish or poultry over them. The three styles we most like to use with them are Pad Thai, teriyaki, and garlicky tomato.

TODD'S FAVORITE STIR-FRIED VEGETABLES

RECIPE BY TODD JOHNSON

2 carrots
1 zucchini, cut in half lengthwise, seeds removed
1 yellow squash, cut in half lengthwise, seeds removed
1 small head of Savoy or Napa cabbage
1 red onion
1 red bell pepper
1 bunch broccoli, destemmed
3 heads baby bok choy
20 snow peas, trimmed (destemmed)
1 tablespoon canola oil
pinch of salt and pepper
soy sauce or teriyaki sauce

Wash all of the vegetables. Thinly cut carrots, zucchini, yellow squash, and savoy or Napa cabbage on an angle, keeping all the cuts the same size.

Cut red onion in half, and julienne thinly. Cut bell pepper in half, deseed, and remove ribs, then julienne thinly. Cut and remove broccoli stems, and finally cut the bottoms of the baby bok choy off and individually remove leaves.

Mix all the vegetables in a container and refrigerate.

Place a pot of salted water and a strainer insert on the stove and bring to a boil. Place a large sauté pan or wok on the stove at high heat. Add all the vegetables to the boiling water and cook for 45 seconds, then remove and shake off excess water. Put the vegetables in the sauté pan or wok and immediately add 1 tablespoon of canola oil. Sauté for 1–2 minutes, tossing the vegetables continuously.

Add soy sauce or teriyaki sauce to taste.

MAKES 4 SERVINGS.

Serving size 8 oz.; Calories 106; Grams fat 1.75; % of calories fat 7; Beta-carotene 9,837 IU; Lutein and zeaxanthin 2,841 mcg; Vitamin C 197 mg; Vitamin E 2.5 IU; Zinc 1.037 mg; Selenium 6.25 mcg; Manganese 0.586 mg

QUICHE PROVENÇALE

RECIPE BY ERIC TRUGLAS AND JOY PURCELL

This quiche is a light lunch or dinner meal, high in beta-carotene, lutein, and zeaxanthin. Serve with mixed green salad and fresh fruit dessert.

8 ounces fresh spinach, destemmed and washed very well, chopped fine (can use frozen spinach, defrosted and squeezed dry)
3 cloves garlic, peeled and minced
½ pound chanterelle mushrooms, sliced (if not available use domestic mushrooms)
3 ripe tomatoes concassé (peeled, deseeded, and diced; see page 229 for instructions. Can use instead low sodium or salt-free canned tomatoes, well drained)
9-inch unbaked, reduced-fat pie shell
3 tablespoons fresh grated Parmesan cheese
¼ cup low-fat Swiss cheese, grated (Do not use preshredded cheese. It is coated and will not melt properly at all.)
1 cup skim milk
¾ cup egg substitute
¼ teaspoon nutmeg
salt and pepper to taste

Preheat oven to 375° F.

In a medium sauté pan sprayed with a nonstick cooking spray, sauté spinach and garlic. Add mushrooms and tomatoes. Turn heat to medium high and reduce the liquid to dry. Cool.

Place vegetable mixture in the bottom of the pie shell.

Layer the cheeses over the vegetable mixture. Toss very lightly.

Combine skim milk, egg substitute, nutmeg, salt and pepper.

Pour egg mixture over vegetables and cheeses.

Bake for 15 minutes, then turn temperature down to 350 degrees. Bake for about 30 minutes more, until the top turns golden. The center should be firm to the touch. Allow quiche to cool slightly until it is warm, not hot.

Slice the warm quiche into 6 pieces.

Garnish with melon and strawberries.

MAKES ONE 9-INCH PIE.

Serving size 1 slice (1/6 of pie); Calories 214; Grams fat 8.2; % of calories fat 34.9; Beta-carotene 3,543 IU; Lutein and zeaxanthin 4,150 mcg; Vitamin C 24 mg; Vitamin E 1 IU; Zinc 1.288 mg; Selenium 7.0 mcg; Manganese 0.472 mg

VEGETARIAN QUESADILLA

RECIPE BY ERIC TRUGLAS

Can be used as an appetizer or snack, or makes an excellent light lunch or dinner.

4 small fat-free flour tortillas
1 cup low-fat cheddar cheese, shredded
3 carrots, thinly sliced, steamed 8–10 minutes
1 head broccoli, chopped, steamed 5–8 minutes
3 papayas, peeled, seeded, and sliced (if not available, use mango)

½ ounce hot salsa
1 teaspoon fresh cilantro, chopped

Heat grill or grill pan on stove.

Preheat oven to 350° F.

Place tortillas on counter. Spread with cheddar, carrots, broccoli, and papaya. Cover each with salsa and fresh cilantro.

Place tortillas on grill to mark tortilla bottom, then fold in half, place on ovenproof plates, and bake for four minutes.

Cool slightly, and cut quesadillas in quarters to serve.

MAKES 4 SERVINGS.

Serving size 1 tortilla; Calories 313; Grams fat 3.443; % of calories fat 10; Beta-carotene 18,396 IU; Lutein and zeaxanthin 2,159 mcg; Vitamin C 247 mg; Vitamin E 9 IU; Zinc 1.178 mg; Selenium 6 mcg; Manganese 0.993 mg

SPINACH QUESADILLA

RECIPE BY ERIC TRUGLAS

An excellent source of beta-carotene, lutein, and zeaxanthin.

4 small fat-free flour tortillas
1 cup low-fat cheddar cheese, shredded
3 cups spinach, chopped, steamed 2–3 minutes
3 papayas, peeled, seeded, and sliced (if not available, use mango)
½ ounce hot salsa
1 teaspoon fresh cilantro, chopped

Heat grill or grill pan on stove.

Preheat oven to 350° F.

Place tortillas on counter. Spread with cheddar, spinach, and papaya. Cover each with salsa and fresh cilantro.

Place tortillas on grill to mark tortilla bottoms then fold

in half, place on ovenproof plates, and bake for 4 minutes. Cool slightly and cut quesadillas in quarters to serve.

MAKES 4 SERVINGS.

Serving size 1 tortilla; Calories 281; Grams fat 7.8; % of calories fat 25; Beta-carotene 2,282 IU; Lutein and zeaxanthin 2,297 mcg; Vitamin C 136 mg; Vitamin E 5 IU; Zinc 1.394 mg; Selenium 5 mcg; Manganese 0.386 mg

SPINACH FETTUCCINE WITH ROASTED PEPPERS AND TOMATOES

RECIPE BY JOY PURCELL

Very easy to put together, because the vegetables are made ahead of time. The sauce is a combination of peppers, shallots, tomatoes, and lots of fresh basil for the garnish. A light and tasty dish, the sauce has a zesty flavor.

1½ pounds plum tomatoes, sliced
2 teaspoons dried basil
1 teaspoon dried oregano
2 teaspoons garlic, finely minced
1 small eggplant (optional)
1 yellow pepper
1 red pepper
1 green pepper
1 small Hungarian wax pepper (These are medium-hot, but have great flavor; be careful to wash hands after handling.)
1 pound spinach fettuccine
1 tablespoon olive oil
4 shallots, peeled and sliced very thin
2 cloves garlic, minced
1 cup strained or crushed tomatoes
4 tablespoons fresh basil, sliced very fine
fresh ground black pepper, to taste

Prepare vegetables for roasting (this may look like a lot of work, but it's actually fairly easy and can be done ahead of time):

Mix tomatoes with the dried basil, dried oregano, and finely minced garlic. Place them on a baking sheet in a 350° F oven and bake until tender. The result is a fresh sauce in which the flavors of the tomatoes and herbs have mingled and become concentrated.

Place whole eggplant on a sheet and bake in the oven. Cool; take the peel off, finely chop, and use as recipe indicates. Eggplant and tomatoes can be done at the same time as they are baked.

Cut peppers in half, and remove the seeds. Place under the broiler or on a gas grill. Let them char and blacken (this will be on the outside only), and cover them so they steam a little. Remove the outer skin, and you will have a pepper that has a great smoky flavor. Roasted peppers splashed with balsamic vinegar make a great appetizer.

Prepare pasta according to directions on package. Keep warm for service.

In a large sauté pan, heat olive oil, then add shallots and garlic. Cook until their aroma rises.

Add the roasted peppers and eggplant, heating through just until hot.

Add the tomatoes to the other ingredients and warm through. Adjust the seasonings.

Serve over the pasta, and garnish with fresh basil.

MAKES 6 SERVINGS.

Serving size 4–6 oz. sauce & 3–4 oz. pasta, cooked; Calories 367; Grams fat 2; % of calories fat 5; Beta-carotene 2,116 IU; Lutein and zeaxanthin 392 mcg; Vitamin C 136 mg; Vitamin E 1 IU; Zinc 2.531 mg; Selenium 1 mcg; Manganese 2.435 mg

VEGETARIAN CASSOULET

RECIPE BY JOY PURCELL

Traditional cassoulet usually has sausage and other meats cooked in with the vegetables to create a rich stew. We have used more vegetables, taken out the meat, and added some wonderful legumes for a healthy alternative. Vary the beans to your choice; these are just suggestions. This dish can be served by itself or with a three-ounce portion of rice, barley, quinoa, or bulgur wheat. Cassoulet is great served with low-fat corn bread.

2 teaspoons olive oil
2 celery stalks, medium diced
1 onion, peeled and medium diced
1 tablespoon garlic, minced
3 carrots, peeled and medium diced
3 tomatoes, peeled, seeded, and diced
2 teaspoons curry powder
1 teaspoon cumin
8 ounces canned black beans, drained
8 ounces canned Great Northern beans, drained
8 ounces canned kidney beans, drained
1–2 cups nonfat vegetable broth
1 red pepper, seeded and diced
1 cup fresh uncooked pumpkin, diced (or use acorn, butternut, turban, or Hubbard squash in place of pumpkin)
½ cup cut corn
1 medium zucchini, diced
1 tablespoon fresh chopped parsley, for garnish
1 tablespoon fresh chopped mint, for garnish
fresh black pepper to taste and for garnish

In an ovenproof pan or baking dish, heat oil and add celery, onion, garlic, and carrots. Sauté until onions are golden brown.

Add tomatoes and heat through.

Add curry powder and cumin and cook for 2 minutes.

Add beans, broth, and the other vegetables, bring liquid to a simmer, cover, and place in a preheated 350° F oven.

Bake until all ingredients are tender, about 40 minutes.

If necessary, place the cassoulet over medium heat, uncovered. Reduce to the proper consistency (liquid should coat the back of a spoon). You may thicken the liquid with a little cornstarch mixed with broth.

Garnish with chopped fresh herbs and black pepper.

MAKES 10 SERVINGS.

Serving size standard vegetarian 6–8 oz.; Calories 135; Grams fat 1.7; % of calories fat 12; Beta-carotene 4,546 IU; Lutein and zeaxanthin 542 mcg; Vitamin C 25 mg; Vitamin E 1 IU; Zinc 0.944 mg; Selenium 5 mcg; Manganese 0.505 mg

Seafood Entrees

GROUPER FLORENTINE

RECIPE BY ERIC TRUGLAS

An excellent source of beta-carotene, vitamin C, and zinc. Good with plain rice or poached or steamed potatoes.

Four 6-ounce grouper fillets (if not available, another white, flaky fish can be substituted)
FILLING:
2 pounds spinach, washed, dried, chopped
4 tablespoons fresh basil, chopped
2 tomatoes, seeded, chopped
salt and pepper
SAUCE:
2 cups nonfat yogurt
2 tablespoons green peppercorns (peppercorns will add spice; reduce the amount of peppercorns as desired to eliminate spice)

Ready steamer with hot water on stove top.

Form pockets in fish fillet by slicing ¾ of the way through.

Combine spinach, basil, tomatoes, and salt and pepper to taste. Stuff grouper fillets with the mixture; place in steamer for 8 to 10 minutes, or until fish is opaque. Remove fish; reserve; keep warm.

Lightly warm yogurt; add peppercorns to taste—the more you add, the spicier the dish will be. Blend in food processor.

To serve, form a circle of yogurt sauce on each of four plates, cut fish fillets in half diagonally, and place on top of sauce.

MAKES 4 SERVINGS.

Serving size 6 oz. grouper portion; Calories 284; Grams fat 2.747; % of calories fat 9; Beta-carotene 15,954 IU; Lutein and zeaxanthin 23,182 ug; Vitamin C 76 mg; Vitamin E 8 IU; Zinc 3.107 mg; Selenium 8 mcg; Manganese 2.160 mg

SALMON EN PAPILLOTE

RECIPE BY ERIC TRUGLAS

Excellent source of beta-carotene, lutein, zeaxanthin, vitamin C, and zinc. Good when served with poached or steamed potatoes, or a mixture of brown and plain rice.

6 medium-size sweet potatoes
1 pound fresh spinach, washed, dried, roughly chopped
1 teaspoon chopped fresh tarragon
1 shallot, chopped
¼ cup (2 ounces) white wine
1 small clove garlic, minced
white pepper
4 pieces papillote (parchment paper) or foil, 8 by 11 inches, folded in half, cut into heart shapes
24 ounces fresh salmon, cut into 4 servings
4 sprigs fresh tarragon

Preheat oven to 375° F.

Place sweet potatoes in small saucepan with water to cover. Bring to boil. When just tender, about 20 minutes, drain, cool, peel, and slice.

Place spinach, tarragon, shallot, and wine in large skillet. Cook over medium heat for 6 to 7 minutes. Add garlic and white pepper to taste, and stir until warmed through. Let cool.

To assemble packets, unfold parchment or foil and place on counter. Divide potatoes and spinach, placing portions in middle of each. Top with salmon and a sprig of tarragon. Fold parchment or foil around food, forming a half-heart again. Crimp edges to seal.

Place packets on a cookie sheet and bake 15 minutes. To serve, place one packet on each dinner plate and open paper a little for steam and the tempting aroma to escape.

MAKES 4 SERVINGS.

Serving size 6-oz. piece of salmon; Calories 499; Grams fat 15.1; % of calories fat 27; Beta-carotene 45,558 IU; Lutein and zeaxanthin 11,591 mcg; Vitamin C 74 mg; Vitamin E 6 IU; Zinc 2.045 mg; Selenium 108 mcg; Manganese 2.087 mg

GRILLED TUNA IN LIGHT SUMMER VINAIGRETTE

RECIPE BY ERIC TRUGLAS

Excellent source of beta-carotene, vitamin C, and magnesium. Good with plain or saffron rice.

VINAIGRETTE:
1 mango or papaya, peeled, seeded, and diced small
1 cup dried apricot
1 cup cantaloupe, diced
1 cup beet greens, chopped (if not available, use other greens)

2 tablespoons fresh cilantro, chopped
2 tablespoons fresh dill, chopped
1 avocado, peeled, pitted, and diced small
1 medium onion, diced small
3 tablespoons chopped basil
1 green, red, or yellow pepper, diced small
1 tablespoon chopped fresh thyme
1 tablespoon olive oil
3 tablespoons fresh lime juice
salt and pepper

MARINADE:
1 tablespoon chopped fresh thyme
1 tablespoon olive oil
3 tablespoons fresh lime juice

4 6-ounce pieces fresh tuna

TO SERVE:
3 cups finely chopped leaf lettuce

Put vinaigrette ingredients in small bowl, mix well, cover, and let stand at room temperature 2 to 3 hours.

In a large shallow bowl, combine ingredients for marinade; place tuna in marinade 15 to 20 minutes; turn occasionally to coat well.

Grill tuna to medium rare (best), or to taste. Keep warm.

To serve, place grilled tuna on plates. Divide lettuce, place to one side, and top all with vinaigrette-marinade mixture.

MAKES 4 SERVINGS.

Serving size 6-oz. piece of tuna; Calories 489; Grams fat 15.816; % of calories fat 29; Beta-carotene 8,141 IU; Lutein and zeaxanthin 226 ug; Vitamin C 86 mg; Vitamin E 5 IU; Zinc 1.839 mg; Selenium 2 mcg; Manganese 0.759 mg

POACHED ATLANTIC SALMON

RECIPE BY TODD JOHNSON

Although this entree has a high fat content, it is mainly omega-3, a type of fat that has been shown to be good for you. The only downside to this meal, as with most meals containing salmon, is the higher calorie content as a result of the "healthy" fat present. Therefore, you should eat salmon with a light side dish or salad to balance out the rich calorie content. This meal goes well with bread, rice, or potato.

1 fillet of salmon
½ cup white wine (e.g., Chardonnay)
1 cup seafood broth or clam juice
1 fresh bay leaf
3 sprigs of thyme
2 whole black peppercorns
3 fresh vine ripe tomatoes, diced
1 teaspoon chopped garlic
2 tablespoons canola oil
4 ounces of fresh spinach

Placc the salmon fillet in a small sauté pan with the wine, seafood broth, bay leaf, thyme, salt to taste, and black peppercorns. Poach the salmon till just translucent in the center. Remove the poaching fluid.

Add the tomatoes to the poaching liquid and cook for 5 minutes, then puree in food processor or blender.

In another sauté pan, lightly brown the garlic in canola oil, then add the spinach; cook for just 1 minute.

Serve the salmon over the spinach; and pour the tomato broth around the salmon. Season with additional pepper to taste.

MAKES 1 SERVING.

Serving size 4–6 oz. salmon with 3 oz. filling; Calories 695; Grams fat 41; % of calories fat 54; Beta-carotene 10,871 IU; Lutein and zeaxanthin 11,591 mcg; Vitamin C 104 mg; Vitamin E 15 IU; Zinc 1.750 mg; Selenium 7 mcg; Manganese 1.964 mg

VEGETABLE AND SHRIMP QUICHE

RECIPE BY ERIC TRUGLAS AND JOY PURCELL

A great appetizer or light lunch, for light dining. Easy to prepare. A good source of beta-carotene and zinc.

1 pound large shrimp, peeled, deveined, cooked, and sliced lengthwise (frozen prepared shrimp may be used)
2 nine-inch unbaked, reduced-fat pie shells
½ cup mushrooms, sliced
2 tablespoons fresh chopped garlic
½ cup fresh or frozen spinach (if you are using fresh spinach you will need to destem and chop)
1 red pepper, seeded and finely diced
1 cup broccoli, cut into small florets and steamed to just tender
1 cup carrots, sliced and cooked to just tender
1 small bunch scallions, diced fine
1 cup egg whites
2 cups skim milk
fresh grated pepper to taste
1 teaspoon Tabasco sauce
1 tablespoon cilantro, finely chopped
2 tablespoons fresh chopped basil
4 tablespoons fresh grated Parmesan cheese

Preheat oven to 375° F.

Place half the shrimp in each pie shell.

In a medium sauté pan cook mushrooms, garlic, and spinach until liquid is gone. Divide into equal parts and place the vegetables over the shrimp into each pie shell. Do the same for the rest of your vegetables.

Mix egg whites, skim milk, herbs, seasonings, and

Parmesan cheese. Pour equal amounts over the vegetable-and-shrimp mix in each pie shell.

Bake for 10–15 minutes, then turn oven down to 350 degrees. Continue to bake for 30 minutes. Pour away any moisture around edges. The filling will be firm to the touch. Cool 10 minutes before cutting into equal pieces. This recipe makes two quiches.

MAKES 16 SERVINGS.

Serving size ⅛ pie; Calories 165; Grams fat 6.004; % of calories fat 33; Beta-carotene 2,917 IU; Lutein and zeaxanthin 377 mcg; Vitamin C 22.96 mg; Vitamin E less than 1 IU; Zinc 0.59 mg; Selenium 21 mcg; Manganese 0.094 mg

SCALLOPS WITH ENDIVE AND DRIED APRICOTS

RECIPE BY ERIC TRUGLAS

An excellent source of beta-carotene and a good source of zinc. Good with steamed potatoes, plain fettuccine, or linguini.

2 teaspoons olive oil
20 jumbo scallops
salt and pepper
6 pieces endive, thinly sliced
2 tablespoons chopped basil
1 cup dried apricots
1 cup apricot juice
fresh basil leaves

Heat olive oil in large skillet. When hot, cook scallops on both sides until opaque (about 20 seconds), then remove from skillet and set aside in a warm place.

In the skillet, braise endive and basil for 2 to 3 minutes, add dried apricots and apricot juice, and cook 4 to 5 minutes.

To serve, put endive and apricot with a little juice in the

middle of each of 4 warm plates. Place 5 scallops around edge. Garnish with basil leaves.

MAKES 4 SERVINGS.

Serving size 5 scallops; Calories 268; Grams fat 1.557; % of calories fat 5; Beta-carotene 4,246 IU; Lutein and zeaxanthin 0 mcg; Vitamin C 8 mg; Vitamin E 3 IU; Zinc 2.128 mg; Selenium 0 mcg; Manganese 0.392 mg

Poultry Entrees

POACHED CHICKEN STUFFED WITH CHANTERELLE MUSHROOMS IN CILANTRO VINAIGRETTE

RECIPE BY ERIC TRUGLAS

A good source of beta-carotene, zinc, and selenium, this is good with mixed steamed vegetables such as carrots, broccoli, cauliflower, and zucchini.

VINAIGRETTE:
3 tablespoons fresh cilantro, chopped
1/8 cup olive oil
2 tablespoons red wine vinegar

12 ounces chanterelle mushrooms, chopped (if not available, use shiitake mushrooms)
1 tablespoon chopped fresh basil
4 5-ounce chicken breasts, skin and fat removed
2 egg whites, beaten
1 teaspoon olive oil

TO FINISH:
3 medium tomatoes, cut in chunks
3 shallots, sliced
1 teaspoon olive oil

GARNISH:
basil leaves or other fresh herbs

Ready a steamer with hot water.

Combine vinaigrette ingredients, cover, and set aside at room temperature.

In a small sauté pan, heat oil. Sauté chanterelle mushrooms and chopped basil for two minutes, and set aside.

To make chicken pieces larger and thinner, pound them carefully with the broad side of a large chef's knife, without cutting through the meat (this is best done by placing chicken breasts between two sheets of waxed paper).

Combine mushroom-basil mixture with beaten egg whites, and cover the chicken breasts with this mixture. Roll chicken in plastic, and secure with twisted ends. Steam 15 minutes. Remove chicken, and set aside in a warm place.

Steam tomatoes two minutes. Meanwhile, sauté shallots in 1 tablespoon olive oil until tender. To serve, unwrap chicken, and cut into medallions (cut across grain of meat to form rounds). Place on four serving plates. Put tomato chunks on top, cover with shallots, spread vinaigrette over all, and add garnish.

MAKES 4 SERVINGS.

Serving size 1 chicken breast; Calories 412; Grams fat 17.5; % of calories fat 38; Beta-carotene 1,359 IU; Lutein and zeaxanthin 83 mcg; Vitamin C 20 mg; Vitamin E 4 IU; Zinc 2.542 mg; Selenium 3 mcg; Manganese 0.285 mg

CHICKEN BREAST STUFFED WITH MONTRACHET GOAT CHEESE, DRIED APRICOTS, AND WATERCRESS

RECIPE BY ERIC TRUGLAS

An excellent source of beta-carotene, and a good source of zinc. This dish goes well with black beans and rice.

4 4-ounce chicken breasts, skin and fat removed.

STUFFING MIXTURE:

3 carrots, very thinly sliced, steamed 12–15 minutes
4 ounces dried apricots
4 ounces Montrachet goat cheese (if not available, use other goat cheese)
3 tablespoons watercress leaves, steamed 12–15 minutes
1 tablespoon chopped garlic
1 tablespoon chopped basil
1 egg yolk
salt and pepper

Preheat oven to 350° F.

Combine all ingredients for stuffing.

Flatten chicken breasts slightly (see the preceding recipe). Place one chicken breast on each of 4 pieces of aluminum foil. Cover each breast with stuffing; roll chicken in foil tightly, twist ends, and place on a baking sheet.

Bake 20 to 25 minutes, then unwrap and slice chicken.

Serve on warm plates.

MAKES 4 SERVINGS.

Serving size 7-ounce chicken breast; Calories 351; Grams fat 6.639; % of calories fat 17.5; Beta-carotene 12,503 IU; Lutein and zeaxanthin 0 ug; Vitamin C 8 mg; Vitamin E 2 IU; Zinc 2.087 mg; Selenium 3 mcg; Manganese 0.217 mg

ROTISSERIE CHICKEN PASTA

RECIPE BY TODD JOHNSON

12 ounces rotisserie chicken meat, in half-inch cubes
12 ounces fettuccine
2 teaspoons olive oil
8 whole sun-dried tomatoes, julienned
2 teaspoons chopped garlic
2 teaspoons chopped shallot
2 ounces raw spinach
8 leaves fresh basil
12 fluid ounces chicken broth
salt and pepper

Precook the chicken meat till done, then refrigerate. (Alternatively, the chicken can be bought at most supermarkets already cooked.) Be sure to remove the skin before using. Precook the fettuccine according to package directions till al dente. Cool with ice water. Add 1 teaspoon olive oil and refrigerate.

Soak the sun-dried tomatoes in warm water for 10 minutes, then strain off water and julienne. Chop the garlic and shallots, and pick the spinach and basil stems. Place a large sauté pan on the stove on medium to high heat. Add 1 teaspoon of olive oil to the pan, along with the minced garlic and shallots. Cook for 2 minutes.

Add the diced chicken meat, sun-dried tomatoes, whole spinach leaves, and basil. Add 6 ounces of chicken broth, then the pasta, and cook till the pasta becomes hot (about 2 minutes). Season with salt and pepper.

MAKES 4 SERVINGS.

Serving size 8 oz. meat & ½ cup sauce; Calories 534; Grams fat 12; % of calories fat 20; Beta-carotene 1,632 IU; Lutein and zeaxanthin 1,449 mcg; Vitamin C 6.5 mg; Vitamin E 1 IU; Zinc 3 mg; Selenium 18.5 mcg; Manganese 0.85 mg

Beef Entrees

CURRIED VEAL

RECIPE BY ERIC TRUGLAS

An excellent source of beta-carotene and zinc, good with plain pasta.

2 ½ pounds cleaned veal loin (can substitute chicken or lamb)
2 teaspoons olive oil
1 onion, chopped
2 tablespoons curry powder
1 teaspoon flour
2 cups fat-free chicken stock
1 clove garlic
6 carrots, diced
½ cup reduced-fat coconut milk
1 tablespoon redcurrant jelly
2 tablespoons skim milk
1 teaspoon arrowroot
6 ripe peaches, peeled and halved

Brown veal slowly in a skillet with half the olive oil.

When brown on all sides, remove from skillet and set aside in a warm place. Heat the remaining olive oil in the skillet, then add onion and let cook for 2 minutes.

Stir in the curry powder and cook 2 minutes. Sprinkle in the flour and cook 1 minute. Remove from heat and pour in the chicken stock. Add garlic. Bring to a boil and simmer 15 minutes.

Return veal to skillet. Add carrots, and cover and cook 35 minutes.

Transfer the veal to a serving platter. Finish the sauce by adding coconut milk and jelly into the skillet. Let simmer 3 minutes, then strain. Stir in the skim milk, and thicken with arrowroot.

Add peaches. Heat sauce and pour over veal.

MAKES 6 SERVINGS.

Serving size slightly less than ½ lb veal; Calories 359; Grams fat 12.176; % of calories fat 32; Beta-carotene 13,648 IU; Lutein and zeaxanthin 0 mcg; Vitamin C 13 mg; Vitamin E 3 IU; Zinc 5.151 mg; Selenium 3 mcg; Manganese 0.399 mg

Sauces

Many sauces or dips are excellent with low-fat chips and crackers, but be careful when you buy chips and crackers, because many packaged foods are made with cooking oils high in saturated fat, which is both fattening and harmful to your blood vessels. However, there are some excellent low-fat choices available, including bagel chips, rice cakes, whole-grain crisp bread, cocktail rye bread, fat-free saltine crackers, wheat crackers, toasted whole-grain pita bread, and homemade sweet or Idaho potato chips.

TOMATILLO SALSA

RECIPE BY ERIC TRUGLAS

This low-fat dip is excellent in combination with toasted pita, sweet potato chips, or bagel chips. It is great served over chicken.

4 tomatillos, outer skin removed and washed (green tomatoes may be substituted)
3 yellow tomatoes, seeded, quartered
1 yellow pepper, diced small
1 yellow onion, peeled and diced
¼ cup chopped scallions
1 teaspoon skinned, seeded, and minced serrano chilis (wash hands well after preparing, as they are very caustic)
½ bunch cilantro leaves, chopped
2 tablespoons red wine vinegar
½ teaspoon ground cumin

Tabasco sauce
salt and black pepper

Mix all ingredients together and let macerate (sit) for 2½ hours. Add Tabasco if you like it more spicy.

MAKES 10 SERVINGS.

Serving size ½ cup; Calories 32; Grams fat 0.292; % of calories fat 8; Beta-carotene 609 IU; Lutein and zeaxanthin 88 mcg; Vitamin C 54 mg; Vitamin E Less than 1 IU; Zinc 0.141 mg; Selenium 1 mcg; Manganese 0.136 mg

TOMATO SALSA

RECIPE BY ERIC TRUGLAS

An excellent dip, rich in beta-carotene, that can also be heated and used as a sauce on pasta.

6 large red tomatoes, seeded and diced fine
1 yellow pepper, diced fine
1 yellow onion, peeled and diced fine
¼ cup chopped scallions
1 teaspoon skinned, seeded, and minced serrano chilis
½ bunch cilantro leaves, chopped fine
2 tablespoons red wine vinegar
½ teaspoon ground cumin
Tabasco sauce
salt and black pepper

Mix all ingredients together and let macerate (sit) for 2½ hours. Add Tabasco if you like it more spicy.

MAKES 4 CUPS (8 SERVINGS).

Serving size ½ cup; Calories 35; Grams fat 0.394; % of calories fat 10; Beta-carotene 653 IU; Lutein and zeaxanthin 200 mcg; Vitamin

C 62 mg; Vitamin E less than 1 IU; Zinc 0.175 mg; Selenium 1 mcg; Manganese 0.157mg

SALSA FRESCA

RECIPE BY TODD JOHNSON

Excellent with low-fat crackers.

4 cups tomato concassé (see instructions below; may substitute canned low-sodium or fat-free tomatoes, well drained)
½ medium red onion, diced small
1 green pepper, diced small
1 red pepper, diced small
½ bunch cilantro, chopped
juice of two limes
½ teaspoon cumin, finely ground
2 jalapeno peppers, finely chopped (Tabasco sauce can be substituted)
1 cup V8 vegetable juice
salt and pepper

To prepare the tomatoes concassé:

Place the tomatoes in a pot of boiling water for 30–60 seconds, then place in ice-cold water. The skin will easily peel off at this point.

Cut the skinless tomatoes in half. Squeeze out the seeds. Dice the remaining tomato pulp.

To complete the dish:

Combine all ingredients, season with salt and freshly ground pepper, and refrigerate until ready to serve.

MAKES 6 CUPS.

Serving size ¼ cup; Calories 13; Grams fat 0.143; % of calories fat 10; Beta-carotene 456 IU; Lutein and zeaxanthin 83 ug; Vitamin C 17 mg; Vitamin E less than 1 IU; Zinc 0.069 mg; Selenium 0 mcg; Manganese 0.058 mg

MANGO AND FRESH HERB COULIS

RECIPE BY ERIC TRUGLAS AND JOY PURCELL

A good source of beta-carotene and vitamin C, goes well with fish or chicken.

3 mangoes peeled, seeded, and cut in chunks
2 shallots, peeled and halved
¼ cup fresh chopped basil
4 drops Tabasco sauce
1 tablespoon fresh mint, finely chopped
white pepper

Purée mangoes and shallots in a blender until smooth. Pour into a medium bowl. Fold in herbs and seasonings. Serve with fish, chicken, or salad. Use a 2-ounce portion.

MAKES 2 CUPS (8 SERVINGS).

Serving size ¼ cup; Calories 53; Grams fat 0.223; % of calories fat 4; Beta-carotene 3,416 IU; Lutein and zeaxanthin 0 mcg; Vitamin C 22 mg; Vitamin E 1 IU; Zinc 0.052 mg; Selenium 1 mcg; Manganese 0.054 mg

Side Dishes

PUREE OF BROCCOLI

RECIPE BY ERIC TRUGLAS AND JOY PURCELL

An excellent source of vitamin C, lutein, and zeaxanthin, good with fish or chicken.

1 pound broccoli, leaves removed, florets and stems cut into large chunks
¼–½ cup evaporated skim milk
salt, pepper, and ground nutmeg

Steam broccoli until tender.

Puree in food processor until smooth, then add skim milk. Taste, and add seasonings. Reheat if necessary. Use a scoop or a baker's piping bag for presentation.

MAKES 2 SERVINGS.

Serving size ½ cup; Calories 65; Grams fat 0.794; % of calories fat 11; Beta-carotene 4,005 IU; Lutein and zeaxanthin 4,318 mcg; Vitamin C 211 mg; Vitamin E 6 IU; Zinc 0.907 mg; Selenium 3 mcg; Manganese 0.521 mg

CARROT PUREE

RECIPE BY ERIC TRUGLAS AND JOY PURCELL

One of my favorites, and an excellent source of beta-carotene and zinc. Excellent with chicken, grouper, snapper, sole, or other white fish.

10 carrots, peeled, cut in large chunks
¼ cup evaporated skim milk
1 teaspoon ground ginger
salt and pepper to taste

Steam carrots until tender.

Puree in food processor until smooth, and add skim milk. Taste, correct seasonings, reheat if necessary. Serve by scooping or piping onto plate.

MAKES 5 SERVINGS.

Serving size ½ cup; Calories 40.92; Grams fat 0.176; % of calories fat 4; Beta-carotene 26,314 IU; Lutein and zeaxanthin 0 mcg; Vitamin C 8 mg; Vitamin E 1 IU; Zinc 0.186 mg; Selenium 2 mcg; Manganese 0.132 mg

CARROTS AU GRATIN

RECIPE BY ERIC TRUGLAS AND JOY PURCELL

An excellent source of beta-carotene, good with beef, lamb, or chicken. Can be made ahead of time and baked at the last minute.

10 carrots, peeled, very thinly sliced
1 tablespoon reduced-fat margarine
2–3 tablespoons shallots or red onions, finely diced
3 cloves garlic, finely diced
1 tablespoon flour
1 cup skim milk
¼ cup low-fat Swiss cheese, grated (Do not use preshredded cheese.)
¼ cup basil, tarragon, or dill
salt and white pepper

Preheat oven to 350° F.

In a large shallow glass baking dish preferably 9 × 9 or similar size, arrange carrots.

Melt the margarine in a small sauté pan. Add shallots and garlic and sauté for 2 minutes. Add flour and stir. This will make a flavorful roux.

Add the milk to the flour mixture and stir until just thickened. Add the cheese to the milk mixture. Stir to melt the cheese. Fold in the herbs and seasonings. Spread over the carrots, making sure the cheese sauce distributes evenly.

Bake for 15–20 minutes, until carrots are tender and the top is golden in color. If the carrots are tender and the top is not golden, place under the broiler for 2–3 minutes or until the top has a golden color.

Cut into 6–8 equal portions and serve.

MAKES 6–8 SERVINGS.

Serving size ⅙ of 9-inch pan; Calories 97; Grams fat 1.512; % of calories fat 14; Beta-carotene 38,254 IU; Lutein and zeaxanthin 289 mcg; Vitamin C 13 mg; Vitamin E less than 1 IU; Zinc 0.658 mg; Selenium 2 mcg; Manganese 0.251 mg

BROCCOLI ALMONDINE

RECIPE BY ERIC TRUGLAS

An excellent source of lutein, zeaxanthin, and vitamin C, this goes well with turkey loin, chicken, or lamb.

1 teaspoon margarine
1 pound fresh broccoli, trimmed and sliced into 2-inch sections
1 tablespoon chopped fresh oregano
freshly ground black pepper
3 tablespoons sliced almonds

In a nonstick skillet, heat the margarine over medium high heat. Add cut broccoli and sauté 2 to 3 minutes, stirring to ensure even cooking.

Add oregano and pepper to taste; sauté 20 to 30 seconds more. Broccoli should be tender-crisp.

Turn into serving dish; sprinkle with almonds; serve immediately.

MAKES 6 SERVINGS.

Serving size ½ cup; Calories 46; Grams fat 2.4; % of calories fat 46; Beta-carotene 1,247 IU; Lutein and zeaxanthin 1,439 mcg; Vitamin C 70 mg; Vitamin E 2 IU; Zinc 0.52 mg; Selenium 0 mcg; Manganese 0.179 mg

OVEN-ROASTED VEGETABLES WITH HERBS AND GARLIC

RECIPE BY JOY PURCELL

A different method of cooking vegetables is to roast them slowly in the oven. The flavors blend, it takes little work, the dish presents very well on the table, and you can use many combinations to satisfy your tastes.

3 carrots, peeled and cut into 1-inch pieces
1 onion, peeled and cut into 1-inch pieces
3 celery stalks, cleaned and cut into 1-inch pieces
1 sweet potato, peeled and cut into 1-inch pieces
1 small leek, washed well, cut into pieces (use the green part also)
2 parsnips, peeled and cut into 1-inch pieces
6 small red potatoes, cut in quarters
6 cloves garlic, peeled and chopped
1 teaspoon dried sage
1 teaspoon dried marjoram
1 teaspoon dried thyme
1 tablespoon nonfat liquid margarine
3 tablespoons fresh chopped parsley

Preheat oven to 375° F.

In a large broiler pan, toss all the ingredients together except the fresh chopped parsley.

Place in the oven and roast slowly until the vegetables are tender but not overcooked. Turn them occasionally to ensure uniform cooking. The vegetables should be lightly browned on the edges. If they are browning too quickly, cover with foil. Cooking time varies, from 30 to 40 minutes.

When the vegetables have finished cooking, place them in a serving bowl or platter and sprinkle with fresh chopped parsley. Fabulous if you use tarragon, rosemary, and chives in place of parsley.

MAKES 4 SERVINGS.

Serving size standard vegetarian 4–6 oz; Calories 203; Grams fat 0.648; % of calories fat 3; Beta-carotene 16,505 IU; Lutein and zeaxanthin 873 mcg; Vitamin C 49 mg; Vitamin E 1 IU; Zinc 1.143 mg; Selenium 3 mcg; Manganese 1.209 mg

QUINOA AND VEGETABLES

RECIPE BY JOY PURCELL

Quinoa is a grain-type product with an interesting texture and quality. Quinoa has to be washed because it contains soaporins, which have a very offensive taste. Fresh vegetables and lime juice are used to give this dish many colors and flavors.

1 cup uncooked quinoa
1 cup cut corn
2 celery stalks, thinly cut on a bias
1 small red pepper, seeded and diced small
2 green onions, diced
1 jalapeño pepper, seeded and minced
1 yellow pepper, seeded and diced small
1/4 cup freshly squeezed key lime juice (regular lime juice will be fine)
fresh ground pepper
1/4 cup fresh chopped parsley
3 tangerines, peeled and segmented

Rinse and cook quinoa according to package directions. Cool and reserve until needed.

Mix vegetables with lime juice.

Toss quinoa with vegetables, seasonings, and parsley. Refrigerate for a couple of hours so the flavors blend. (If the quinoa salad needs salt, try adding a little lemon juice or Tabasco sauce.)

Serve on a platter, on a bed of green leafy vegetables, and surround with the tangerine segments.

MAKES 8 SERVINGS.

Serving size 1 cup; Calories 125; Grams fat 1.521; % of calories fat 11; Beta-carotene 616 IU; Lutein and zeaxanthin 700 mcg; Vitamin C 71 mg; Vitamin E less than 1 IU; Zinc 0.969 mg; Selenium 1 mcg; Manganese 0.581 mg

Desserts

EXOTIC FRUIT TARTE

RECIPE BY ERIC TRUGLAS

Excellent source of beta-carotene and vitamin C.

2 mangoes, diced
2 papayas, diced
½ pineapple, diced
4 kiwis, diced
2 carambola (star fruit), diced
4 figs, diced
4 passion fruit, diced
4 ounces sugar
1 ounce rum
4 4 × 6 phyllo dough leaves (used for baklava)
½ cup fresh mint, chopped

In a preheated skillet simmer all of the fruit for 5 minutes, then add sugar and rum. Let simmer 8 more minutes, then let cool.

Cut phyllo dough into 8 rectangular sheets and bake.

To serve, place phyllo dough sheet in the center of a plate, pour some of the fruit on top of it, and place another phyllo sheet on top.

Garnish with mint and fresh passion fruit.

MAKES 8 SERVINGS.

Serving size 1 slice of tart; Calories 277; Grams fat 1.658; % of calories fat 5; Beta-carotene 2,874 IU; Lutein and zeaxanthin 0 mcg; Vitamin C 126 mg; Vitamin E 4 IU; Zinc 0.346 mg; Selenium 2 mcg; Manganese 0.739 mg

LAYERED FRUIT PARFAIT

RECIPE BY JOY PURCELL

Light, fresh, and eye-appealing, this dessert is for summer dinners. Layered in a tall stemmed glass, the look is elegant and easy to prepare.

1 pint fresh strawberries, washed and cut into pieces
2 cups nonfat vanilla yogurt
2 cups fresh cantaloupe, diced
1 pint fresh raspberries, washed
1 orange, cut into quarters

You will need four white wine glasses rubbed with a little orange peel around the rim. Dip the rim of the glass in sugar to create a very nice garnish for the glass.

Divide the strawberries equally among all the glasses, placing them in the bottom of each glass.

Layer 2 ounces of yogurt over the strawberries in each glass; try to cover the fruit.

Do the same with the diced cantaloupe, ½ cup per glass.

Layer one more time with yogurt, then finish off with the raspberries in each glass.

Make a cut between the orange and the peel about an inch and a half. Do this for all four orange segments. This is your garnish. Slip the cut side onto the glass, flesh side facing out.

MAKES 4 SERVINGS.

Serving size 4 oz. yogurt with 8 oz. fruit; Calories 149; Grams fat 0.735; % of calories fat 4; Beta-carotene 2,734 IU; Lutein and zeaxanthin 0 mcg; Vitamin C 86 mg; Vitamin E less than 1 IU; Zinc 1.581 mg; Selenium 2 mcg; Manganese 0.775 mg

POACHED PEACHES WITH ZINFANDEL STRAWBERRY SAUCE

RECIPE BY JOY PURCELL

Peaches have a delicate flavor when poached in wine and cinnamon. Drizzled with a fresh strawberry coulis, the tastes are exquisite. This is a healthy dessert that looks as great as it tastes. It looks best if served in champagne glasses (not the fluted kind, but the shorter, more saucer-shaped type).

6 peaches, blanched in boiling water for about 30 seconds to remove skins (cut in half and remove pits)
1 cup red Zinfandel (Merlot or Beaujolais will work)
2 ounces mixed berry jelly
¼ cup orange juice
1 stick cinnamon
2 whole cloves
1 pint strawberries, washed, trimmed, and halved
6 mint sprigs

In a saucepan, combine the peaches with Zinfandel, jelly, and orange juice.

Put the cinnamon and cloves in cheesecloth, tie it and place with the peaches. Called a sachet bag, it is used to keep particles from getting into the sauce.

Place the saucepan over medium heat and simmer the peaches for about 10 minutes or until fruit is just tender. Remove the sachet bag and discard.

Remove peaches and chill.

Add the strawberries to the poaching liquid and just heat through. Place the strawberries with liquid into a blender; puree to a smooth consistency.

Strain the strawberry sauce through a fine sieve to remove seeds. Push as much of the fruit pulp through as you can. If at this point the sauce is a little watery, thicken with cornstarch mixed with a little Zinfandel. Bring to a simmer and add the cornstarch mixture, stirring constantly until thick and clear.

Place peach halves in the glass, ladle strawberry sauce over them, and garnish with the mint sprig.

MAKES 6 SERVINGS.

Serving size 1 peach with 2–3 oz. sauce; Calories 94; Grams fat 0.198; % of calories fat 2; Beta-carotene 557 IU; Lutein and zeaxanthin 0 mcg; Vitamin C 25 mg; Vitamin E 1 IU; Zinc 0.213 mg; Selenium 2 mcg; Manganese 0.187 mg

APPENDIX 1

Name Brand and Generic Sunglass Lens Selection

I have tested a number of sunglasses to determine how well they will protect you from macular degeneration. The results are listed in Appendix 2, and are discussed below. The name of the manufacturer is listed first, followed by the lens color and/or type, then by the amount of UVB, UVA, blue, visible, and infrared light transmitted by the lens. The lens material is also listed.

Originally I included lens quality, but, owing to the subjective nature of the testing, I have deleted it. In general, I found that the more expensive name-brand sunglasses had better optical quality than the generic lenses, and glass lenses typically did better than plastic. Briko, Calvin Klein, Cebe, Gargoyles, Hobie, Oakley, Ray-Ban, Revo, and Vuarnet all make excellent-quality lenses.

After buying and testing a wide selection of lenses, I contacted the major manufacturers to see if they had lenses that met my criteria that I had missed. Revo, Oakley, Hobie, Ray-Ban, and Gargoyles were very helpful in providing additional pairs for testing and providing information. Vuarnet provided additional information, but I never received a return phone call from Bolle. As a result, for the manufacturers who responded, I have more information.

The following section is intended to help simplify the task of understanding the results.

How to Select an Inexpensive Lens

Perhaps you are one of those people who just can't help losing their sunglasses, and you do not want to spend a lot of money on a pair of sunglass lenses. Three of the less expensive sunglass lenses provided excellent protection (Fairwind red lens, Family Optic SportsEssentials gray with blue mirror, and the Solar Shield amber lens). Unfortunately, knowing what you are getting when you buy inexpensive sunglasses is difficult. When you go to a store such as Wal-Mart or Kmart, or to the supermarket or drugstore, you'll find the sunglasses on racks, and generically labeled. In other words, unlike Oakley, Gargoyles, Revo, Hobie, or Vuarnet, with which each frame and each type of lens has a specific name, so that you know exactly what you are getting, inexpensive sunglasses do not. Fortunately, there is one exception, amber-colored Solar Shields, which I tested from more than one source. They provided excellent protection, though I did not like the color, which did produce some color distortion. Nevertheless, for ten to fifteen dollars, the lens affords excellent protection.

How to Select a Name Brand

The companies making sunglasses for sports tend to have the ones that give the best protection. These include Adidas, Bolle, Briko, Cebe, Hobie, Oakley, Ray-Ban, Revo, and Vuarnet.

Although many of those manufacturers make sunglasses that met my criteria, leading you to the same sunglasses I tested is not always easy. For Oakley, Revo, Vuarnet, Gargoyles, Ray-Ban, and Hobie I have figured out how to do it. The information you will need is under the section on each manufacturer.

You are probably wondering which is best. This is not an easy question to answer, as each of the manufacturers has advantages, and what may be best for one use may not be ideal for another. Start with the ones that provide the protection you need, and make your selection from that group depending on how they fit you, your lifestyle, and your sense of style.

For sports, Oakley, Hobie, Gargoyles, and Revo provide excellent protection, as do Revo and Hobie for use on the water. For skiing, Vuarnet is excellent, although the lenses are glass, which is not ideal. For driving and day-to-day use, Oakley, Revo, Gargoyles, and Hobie are best. For those who have a hard time with dark sunglasses, Revo's lighter lenses provide excellent protection.

Certain manufacturers have proprietary technology that makes their lenses unique. Revo has a special coating process, Gargoyles a special curvature, and Hobie a special polarization process. We will learn more about these in the section on each manufacturer.

Gargoyles

This company makes one lens that meets my criteria, the gold lens (which transmitted 12% of visible light). The silver lens (transmitted 12%) also provides great protection; it just lets in a little too much blue (8%) and UVB (1%). The gold lens is the only one with a gold mirror, and the silver lens the only one with a silver mirror. Both lenses are polycarbonate, and they are available in the Classics, Legends, Legends II, and Paladin styles; the silver lens also comes in the Helios style.

Gargoyles sunglasses became well known for the curvature of their lens, designed to match the curvature of the cornea and the rotation of the eye. This is reported to reduce the prismatic effect of the lens, which is the tendency of lenses to move the image of what you see so that it is not exactly where you see it. If you were to look at a clock in front of you and you placed a prism in front of you, it would give you the impression the clock had moved to the right, left, up, or down or was turned at an angle, depending on how you held the prism. Typically, we adapt quickly to these changes, but for sports and other activities, eliminating this prismatic effect may enable you to interact with the surrounding environment more effectively. In comparison, most other manufacturers produce their wrap lenses so that the center of the lens is in the center of your head, not the center of your eye. The result is prismatic distortion. While in theory this sounds important, I have not found that it makes a great deal of difference in my testing.

Because of the built-in curvature, you cannot get a Gargoyle prescription lens. They do, however, make the classic frame with a second inner frame or insert into which you can put your prescription glasses to make, in effect, a pair of prescription sunglasses.

Giorgio Armani

If fashion is your objective, Giorgio Armani makes an excellent lens for protection and comfort. As is the case with so many sunglass lenses, when you buy an Armani, you can never be sure exactly which lens you are getting in the glasses you select—or at least that was what I found in my tests of the retail outlets.

Hobie

Hobie makes seven different polarized sunglass lenses at the time of this writing. Four are glass, two are CR39 (plastic), and one is acetate. I tested the CR39s, the gray glass, and the acetate lenses. The copper CR39 (10%) met all but my UV light transmission criteria, letting in 1% of UVB, which is too much. The gray CR39 (8%) and gray glass (8%) did better, but let in a little too much blue light (7% and 6%, respectively) to meet my criteria. The gray acetate (8%) provided the best protection and met all my criteria. It is the only lens they use in the shield and the ultra shield, so if you buy one of these frames, you will know you are getting the right lens. Since the only plastic lenses Hobie uses in its other frames are the CR39 copper and CR39 gray lenses, if you select one of the other frames with gray or copper plastic lenses you will know you are getting these lenses.

Hobies were invented by Hobie Aster, who created a better surfboard in the 1950s. Ten years later he imagined a sailboard that even beginners would have fun with, and from that came the Hobie Cat, one of the world's most popular sailboards. With the same sense of innovation, Aster opened a sunglass lens company in 1983. His glasses all feature a polarized film to help block glare from asphalt, ice, and water.

OAKLEY

Oakley made seven types of lenses the last time I checked: Black iridium (transmitted 8% of visible light), gold iridium (11%), red iridium (15%), gray (24%), VR 28 (28%), high-intensity yellow (88%), and clear (92%). All the lenses are polycarbonate. The gold iridium lens is the only Oakley lens that meets my criteria, and it is the one to ask for. When you buy a pair of Oakley sunglasses, you can specify which type of lens you want, and most salespeople will know what you are talking about. Just in case they don't, gold iridium lenses are the only Oakleys with a gold mirror lens.

You can get the gold iridium lens in any frame type, so once you decide on the frame, all you have to do is tell them you want it with this lens. If they don't have it, they should be able to order it.

If you don't like the gold iridium lens, and are set on a pair of Oakleys, the black iridium is a close second. Although it lets in more than 5% of blue light (the value was 6%), it otherwise meets all the criteria and affords excellent protection for those who prefer gray lenses. If you are playing golf, and there is not much reflected light, but you still want some protection, you can select one of the other lenses that allow even more light in.

The sunglass test results table (Apendix 2) includes the results of three Oakley sunglasses that, as far as I am aware, are no longer made: the gray, amber with gold mirror, and the green with violet mirror. The test results are included in case you should come across them.

Ray-Ban

Like Oakley, Ray-Ban makes great sunglass lenses, with excellent optical quality and frames. Unfortunately, Ray-Ban lenses fell just a hair short of my selection criteria on the amount of visible light, blue light, UVA they transmitted. The best pair, the Daddy O square wrap (10%), did not make the cut for blue light (9.6%) transmission and allowed 1% of UVA, but it came close and is otherwise a good lens. If you are in love with Ray-Ban lenses, their gray polarized lens offers the best protection (this is the lens in the Daddy O square wrap). It does come in other frame types, specifically the Predator and the Daddy O oval wrap. In fact, it is the only gray polarized lens in these frame types, so if it says it's polarized, and it's gray, and it's in these frames, then that is what you are getting.

Ray-Ban's history, like Revo's and Gargoyles', is interesting. In 1951, in response to a Navy Air Corps requirement, Bausch & Lomb, the manufacturer of Ray-Ban glasses, developed what they called a truly neutral sunglass lens, the N-15 (which transmits 15% of visible light). The lens was reengineered for prescription use and renamed the G-15. The military was so satisfied that it wrote an entire set of specifications around the lens. The G-15 is designed to let in more light in the green and yellow portion of the visible light spectrum, because the eye is more sensitive to these colors than to blue or red. Strip clubs use red light because you cannot see as clearly with red light as with the shorter wavelengths, and the eye is less sensitive to it. This covers up blemishes and so on that you might otherwise see. By letting in more of the colors the eye is most sensitive to, theoretically such a lens helps you see better. For military operations such as bombing missions, this is important, and the G-15 works well. In addition, by reducing light transmission to 15%, it preserves night vision, so pilots have optimal vision for night missions as well. When protection is the goal, however, the G-15 is not the best lens.

Revo

Of the lenses I tested, Revo's Stealth glass polarized lens (transmits 12% visible light) is one of the best in terms of the balance between protection and comfort, while providing excellent clarity. If you do not like polarized lenses, the regular Stealth lens (12%) and the gold lens (11%) provide similar protection.

The five Revo lens types I tested were the gold (11%), Stealth (12%), green mirror (13%), blue (14–15%), and the neutral (15%) lenses. The way to identify the blue lens is by its blue color; the Stealth has a silver mirror with a slight blue tint; the gold has a gold coating; the neutral does not have an iridescent coating; and the green lens has a green mirror.

The lenses come in up to three types, glass, glass polarized, and polycarbonate. The sunglasses with glass lenses are the Revo series. The sunglasses with polarized glass lenses are the H2O series, and those with polycarbonate lenses are the Icon series. The blue lens, which is available in all three lens types, looks the same in all three (glass, polycarbonate, and polarized glass) and provides similar amounts of protection in each.

Revo is the only manufacturer that uses lens coating technology to achieve the optimal protection for your eyes. Originally developed by NASA and used to coat space-based optical devices such as the Hubbell Space Telescope, these coatings, unlike those on most sunglasses, are applied in a unique way to block such specific types of light as UV, blue, and infrared. Because of this technology, which is called the Light Management System™ (LMS™), it is the only company that provided excellent protection from blue light across all the lenses I tested. If you find a transmission of 12% or less too dark, picking a lighter Revo lens is an excellent choice and will provide you with some of the best protection you can buy in a lighter lens.

Revo is well known not only for the optical quality but for the camera quality of its lenses. It also polishes its polarized lenses on all four surfaces. Polarized lenses are made by sandwiching a thin plastic film between two pieces of plastic. Most manufacturers polish only two of the surfaces.

Vuarnet

Vuarnet lenses are well labeled, and if you request the Skilynx (7%), polarized PX3000 (5%), or Unilynx (8%), you will get excellent protection. Although I did not test them, according to material I received the PX5000 (4%), polarized PX2000 (5%), and brown polycarbonate lenses (12%) also provide great protection. The brown polycarbonate lenses are available in frames for children. All but the brown polycarbonate lenses are glass, which is not ideal for sports, and all but the brown polycarbonate lens are too dark to meet the ANSI requirements for use while driving. The blue light transmission is below my 2% target on the Skilynx and the Unilynx, which means they induce color distortion.

APPENDIX 2

Sunglass Test Results

Brand/Style	Lens Color	UVB Trans	UVA Trans	Blue Light Transmission	Visible Light Transmission	Infrared Transmission	Lens Material
Adidas A115	gray with silver mirror	0	0	5	9	25	plastic
Adidas A234	brown	0	0	2	8	100	plastic
Adidas Condor2	gray with silver mirror	0	0	7	11	35	plastic
Adidas Gale Force (ski goggle)	gray with blue mirror	0	0	5	6	cannot test	plastic
Adidas Hooker	gray with gold mirror	0	0	3	8	25	plastic
Adidas Wasp	gray	0	0	9	12	50	plastic
Arnette Catfish	amber	0	0	2	13	35	plastic
Arnette Dogs	gray polarized	0	2	10	10	18	glass
Arnette Mantis	gray	0	0	7	11	100	plastic
Arnette Optic Illusions	green	0	2	9	12	0	glass
Arnette Threat	gray	0	0	8	13	100	plastic
Blue Blockers	amber	0	2	3	20	70	plastic
Bluemax	brown-orange	1	1	0	8	100	plastic

Sunglass Test Results *(cont.)*

Brand/Style	Lens Color	UVB Trans	UVA Trans	Blue Light Transmission	Visible Light Transmission	Infrared Transmission	Lens Material
Bolle 450 Geometric	brown	0	0	2	14	35	plastic
Bolle 473 Geometric	green-black	0	0	4	9	25	plastic
Bolle Opsis	gray with blue mirror	0	0	5	10	50	plastic
Bolle 400	gray polarized	0	3	12	12	9	glass
Bolle 426	brown polarized	0	3	9	18	100	glass
Bolle Acryles 527	gray polarized	0	0	15	24	100	plastic
Bolle Acrylex 527	gray with blue mirror	0	0	10	13	35	plastic
Bolle Acrylex 527	amber with gold mirror	0	0	0	4	50	plastic
Bolle Action Sport Breakaway	gray with blue mirror	0	0	4	11	35	plastic
Bolle Action Sport Breakaway	yellow	1	0	36	92	100	plastic
Bolle Action Sport Breakaway	brown	0	0	0	10	35	plastic
Bolle Action Sport Breakaway	orange	0	0	11	38	100	plastic

Bolle Action Sport Breakaway	light amber	0	0	18	45	71	plastic
Bolle Action Sport Breakaway	clear	0	0	64	95	100	plastic
Bolle Action Sport Breakaway	dark gray	0	0	6	13	35	plastic
Bolle Action Sport Breakaway	light gray	0	0	10	18	35	plastic
Bolle Eagle Vision II	gray	0	0	14	24	50	plastic
Briko B-Zone Sporteyes	green with gold mirror	0	0	5	11	100	plastic
Briko Sporteyes Shot Traditional	rose	0	0	32	51	100	plastic
Briko Sporteyes Shot Traditional	brown	0	0	1	8	100	plastic
Briko Stinger Classic	amber (thramamatic)	0	0	9	26	100	plastic
Briko Stinger Classic	green with violet mirror	0	0	3	9	100	plastic
Briko Stinger Classic	brown green with blue mirror	0	0	2	8	100	plastic

Sunglass Test Results *(cont.)*

Brand/Style	Lens Color	UVB Trans	UVA Trans	Blue Light Transmission	Visible Light Transmission	Infrared Transmission	Lens Material
Bucci Airlite Oval	brown with blue mirror	0	0	0	7	0	glass
Bucci Beta	gray	0	1	11	16	9	glass
Bucci Cat	brown polarized	0	0	2	8	18	glass
Bucci the Curve	gray	0	1	9	13	9	glass
Cabbage Patch Kids/Wal-Mart	gray	0	0	6	13	50	plastic
Calvin Klein 139S	brown	0	0	7	14	100	plastic
Calvin Klein 222S	brown	0	0	5	18	6	glass
Calvin Klein 235S	brown	0	0	5	19	6	glass
Calvin Klein 240S	gray	0	0	7	14	100	plastic
Calvin Klein 332S	green	0	2	9	12	0	glass
Calvin Klein 617S	gray	0	0	7	14	100	plastic
Cebe 09350043	green	0	0	3	11	0	glass
Cebe 17810114	brown with blue mirror	0	0	0	7	35	plastic
Crown Polaroid Wal-Mart	amber	0	0	5	17	70	plastic
Crown Polaroid Wal-Mart	light amber	0	0	6	20	70	plastic

Fairwind	blue	0	6	49	13	100	plastic
Fairwind	red	0	0	0	9	70	plastic
Family Optics Beach Essentials	gray	0	2	12	16	50	plastic
Family Optics Men's Fashion	brown gradient	0	0	10 to 24	26 to 45	100	plastic
Family Optics Men's Fashion	gray gradient	0	4 to 9	6	6 to 26	100	plastic
Family Optics Sports Essentials	gray with blue mirror	0	0	1	3	35	plastic
Florence Line Vogue Luxottica Group	gray with black mirror	0	0	5	7	50	plastic
Florence Line Vogue Luxottica Group	green with black mirror	0	1	6	9	4–6	glass
Foster Grant Wal-Mart	brown	0	1	4	14	70	plastic
Gargoyles	dark green	0	0	12	23	50	plastic
Gargoyles	gray	1	0	9	17	35	plastic
Gargoyles	gray with silver mirror	1	0	8	12	25	plastic
Gargoyles	Black Ice (gray)	1	0	11	12	50	plastic
Gargoyles	gold	0	0	5	12	50	plastic

Sunglass Test Results *(cont.)*

Brand/Style	Lens Color	UVB Trans	UVA Trans	Blue Light Transmission	Visible Light Transmission	Infrared Transmission	Lens Material
Giorgio Armani Luxottica Group	green	0	0	4	8	0	glass
Giorgio Armani Luxottica Group	brown	0	0	3	12	0	glass
Gitano Wal-Mart	brown	0	0	4	14	35	plastic
Hobie Sunglasses Elite Pico	dark gray polarized	0	0	6	8	18	glass
Hobie Sunglasses Litroshield	dark gray polarized—acetate	0	0	5	8	100	plastic
Hobie Sunglasses Eclipse	dark gray polarized CR39	0	0	7	11	25	plastic
Hobie Sunglasses Durango	Copper CR-39	1	0	3	10	71	plastic
IREX	Anodized Copper 3000	0	0	0	9	18	plastic
Island Shades	light gray	0	0	12	21	50	polycarbonate
Killer Loop Bausch & Lomb	gray with blue mirror	0	0	12	15	100	plastic

Oakley	gray	0	0	16	19	100	plastic
Oakley	amber with gold mirror	0	0	0	3	12	plastic
Oakley	green with violet mirror	0	0	8	18	100	plastic
Oakley M Frame	red iridium (gray)	0	0	13	15	25	plastic
Oakley Straight Jacket	black iridium (gray)	0	0	6	8	35	plastic
Oakley Topcoat	gold iridium (brown)	0	0	3	11	25	plastic
Optic Nerve	light green	0	0	47	69	100	plastic
Panama Jack	brown	0	0	4	15	65	plastic
Petite Miss Wal-Mart	gray	0	1	7	9	70	plastic
Ray-Ban Gatsby deluxe2	gray-15	0	0	7	13	12	glass
Ray-Ban Driving	Chromax Yellow	0	0	7	23	100	plastic
Ray-Ban Sidestreet	gray, polarized	0	1	8	17	71	plastic
Ray-Ban Rituals	brown	0	1	5	19	35	plastic
Ray-Ban Sidestreet	gray/green	0	1	13	17	25	plastic
Ray-Ban Daddy O	gray polarized	0	1	9	10	18	plastic
Revo H2O	polarized Stealth (brown with silver mirror)	0	0	4	12	0	glass
Revo H2O	polarized blue (brown with blue mirror)	0	0	4	15	9	glass

Sunglass Test Results *(cont.)*

Brand/Style	Lens Color	UVB Trans	UVA Trans	Blue Light Transmission	Visible Light Transmission	Infrared Transmission	Lens Material
Revo H20	polarized neutral (brown, no mirror)	0	0	5	15	35	glass
Revo	Stealth (brown with silver mirror)	0	0	3	12	9	glass
Revo	green (brown with gold mirror)	0	0	3	11	6	glass
Revo	gold (brown with green mirror)	0	0	2	13	4	glass
Revo	neutral (brown with no mirror)	0	0	3	15	0	glass
Revo	blue (brown with blue mirror)	0	0	2	14	0	glass
Revo Icon Upsweep	blue (brown with blue mirror)	0	0	3	14	35	polycarbonate
Solar Shield	amber	0	0	0	9	35	plastic
Solar Shield Wal-Mart	amber	0	0	0	9	35	plastic

Solar SPEX Wal-Mart	orange	0	0	0	29	100	plastic
Solar SPEX Wal-Mart	green/black	0	1	19	18	100	plastic
Solbronze	pink	0	16	42	20	100	plastic
Solbronze	purple	0	33	60	26	100	plastic
Vuarnet PX 2000	brown	0	0	3	16	9	glass
Vuarnet Skilynx	brown	0	0	0	7	12–25	glass
Vuarnet PX3000	polarized gray	0	0	2	5	0	glass
Vuarnet Unilynx	brown	0	0	0	8	18	glass

Appendix 3

What to Know About Prescription Sunglasses

When it comes to getting the ideal amount of protection from a pair of prescription sunglasses, there is no way to know what you are getting at most optical shops. The best way to get the protection you need is to buy one of the lenses I have tested that meet or exceed my guidelines from a name-brand manufacturer.

Although this seems as though it should be easy, it is not. Many optical outlets are not set up to allow you to order prescription sunglass lenses from the major brand-name suppliers. In Florida, for example, only one of the eleven Sunglass Hut outlets was set up for the sale of prescription sunglasses at the time of this writing. Fortunately, if you can't find an outlet to order your sunglasses, you can get some of them directly from the manufacturer. All you need is information from the last shop that made your prescription glasses.

The three companies that make the best prescription sunglasses are Oakley, Revo, and Vuarnet. You can also order from Hobie and Ray-Ban, which make great lenses that just do not meet all my guidelines. Though these manufacturers do not make inexpensive prescription sunglasses, at least you will know what you are getting, because they will have excellent optical quality, and the frames will be well made.

Under each manufacturer you will find a brief review of the lenses that meet, or come closest to meeting, my guidelines. Once you have picked out a lens, you will need to select a frame. Most frames work with prescription sunglass lenses, with the exception of wraparound frames. These frames, owing to the curvature of the lenses used, are not available as prescription sunglasses. If you want side protection, it is best achieved by selecting frames with thick, wide temples.

Prescription Sunglass Lens Review by Manufacturer

Bolle

I understand Bolle makes prescription sunglasses to order, but as of this writing I have been unable to get direct verification of this. If I have difficulty, you are likely to have difficulty as well. Bolle does make some lenses that provide excellent protection; the only problem is that I do not and have not been able to find out how you order them.

Hobie

Hobie makes two plastic lenses; of these, the CR39 gray lens provides the better protection, although neither met my guidelines. The CR39 gray lens lets in a little too much blue light, and the brown CR39 copper lens lets in a little too much UV light, but they otherwise met my guidelines. I did not test all four types of glass lenses they make, but they make copper and gray glass lenses that are reported to have transmission characteristics similar to the plastic ones I tested. Hobie lenses can be ordered to correct for astigmatism (up to 4 diopters) and for moderately strong prescriptions (– 6.00 to +6.00 diopters).

IREX

One of the best manufacturers of prescription sunglass lenses used to be IREX. For years they supplied Bolle with their sunglass lenses, but Bolle now makes its own lenses. IREX lenses are polycarbonate, so they are safe and result in one of the thinnest plastic prescription lenses possible. They employ technology developed by NASA for use on the Apollo space missions. The only IREX available is the Anodized Copper 3000 lens, which provides excellent protection. Its only drawback is that it exceeds my recommended amount of blue light protection, which results in color distortion. It blocks 100% of UVA and UVB, and lets in only 9% of visible light. Unfortunately, IREX is under new management, and has decided not to make any new lenses. There are still some available, but the supplies are going fast. If you don't mind the color distortion, this lens provides excellent protection. You can find out where to get them by calling (800) 500-IREX.

Oakley

Oakley's gold iridium lens provides excellent protection, and can be ordered in a prescription lens. So can the black iridium, which is almost as good, but slightly exceeds my blue light transmission target. They are only available for people who are mildly nearsighted (–4.00 or less diopters) or farsighted (+2.00 or less diopters).

Ray-Ban

Ray-Ban makes a gray polarized lens that provides good protection, but does not quite meet all my guidelines: it lets in a little too much UVA light and blue light. If you prefer a Ray-Ban lens, however, this is the one to get.

Revo

Revo's nonpolarized Stealth lens is available as a prescription sunglass lens. It provides excellent protection and meets all of my criteria. Its only drawback is that it is glass, which means it is not ideal for sports.

Vuarnet

Vuarnet makes three lenses that provide excellent protection and are available as prescription lenses: the Skilynx, unilynx, and the PX3000. They are not available for people who are very farsighted (greater than +5.00 diopters), very nearsighted (less than –5.00 diopters), or those who need correction of an astigmatism. I tested two of the lenses, the Skilynx and Unilynx. I did not test the PX3000. The PX3000 should provide excellent protection, according to the information Vuarnet sent me. Drawbacks of these lenses are they are too dark to meet the ANSI guidelines for use while driving; they are glass, which means they are not ideal for sports; and the Unilynx and Skilynx transmit less than 2% of blue light, which means they induce color distortion.

WHOM TO CALL

Mail-order numbers

Hobie	(800) 283-6938
Oakley	www.oakley.com

Retail Outlet Information

Bausch and Lomb/Ray-Ban/Revo	(800) 343-5594
Hobie	(800) 554-4335
IREX	(800) 500-IREX
Oakley	(800) 403-7449
Vuarnet	(800) 348-0388

References

General References

Basic and clinical science course. 1992. San Francisco: American Academy of Ophthalmology.

Berger, J. W., S. L. Fine, and M. Maguire. 1999. *Age-Related Macular Degeneration.* 1st ed. St. Louis, Mo.: Mosby.

Gass, J. D. 1997. *Stereoscopic Atlas of Macular Diseases, Diagnosis and Treatment.* 4th ed. St. Louis, Mo.: Mosby.

Tasman, W., and E. A. Jaeger. 1998. *Duane's Clinical Ophthalmology.* Philadelphia: J. B. Lippincott Company.

Yanoff, M., and B. S. Fine. 1989. *Ocular Pathology, a Text and Atlas.* 3d ed. Grand Rapids, Michigan: J. B. Lippincott Company.

Chapter 2: How Macular Degeneration Develops

NEW AND EXPERIMENTAL TREATMENTS

DeJuan, E., and R. Machemer. 1998. "Vitreous Surgery for Hemorrhagic and Fibrous Complications of Age Related Macular Degeneration." *American Journal of Ophthalmology* 15:215.

Figueroa, M.S., A. Regueras, and J. Bertrand. 1994. "Laser Photocoagulation to Treat Macular Soft Drusen in Age-Related Macular Degeneration." *Retina* 14:391–396.

Machemer, R., and U. H. Steinhorst. 1993. "Retinal Separation, Retinotomy, and Macular Relocation: II. A Surgical

Approach for Age Related Macular Degeneration." *Graefe's Archive of Clinical Experimental Ophthalmology* 231:635–641.

Miller, J. 1998. "An Update on Photodynamic Therapy." *Review of Ophthalmology* 5, no. 7: 92–94.

Thomas, A. T., J. D. Dickinson, N. S. Melberg et al. 1994. "Visual Results After Surgical Removal of Subfoveal Choroidal Neovascular Membranes." *Ophthalmology* 101:1384–1396.

Chapter 3: Understanding the MD Risk Factors

LACK OF ANTIOXIDANTS

Eye Disease Case-Control Study Group. 1993. "Antioxidant Status and Neovascular Age-Related Macular Degeneration." *Archives of Ophthalmology* 111:104–109.

Eye Disease Case-Control Study Group. 1992. "Risk Factors for Neovascular Age-Related Macular Degeneration." *Archives of Ophthalmology* 110:1701–1708.

Goldberg, J., G. Flowerdew, E. Smith et al. 1988. "Factors Associated with Age-Related Macular Degeneration." *American Journal of Epidemiology* 128:700–710.

TOBACCO SMOKING AND HEAVY ALCOHOL CONSUMPTION

Klein, B. E. K., and R. Klein. 1993. "Cigarette Smoking and Lens Opacities: The Beaver Dam Eye Study." *American Journal of Preventive Medicine* 9:27–30.

Seddon, J. M., W. C. Willett, F. E. Speizer, and S. E. Hankinson. 1996. "A Prospective Study of Cigarette Smoking and Age-Related Macular Degeneration in Women." *Journal of the American Medical Association* 276:1141–1146.

Smith, W., P. Mitchell, and S. R. Leeder. 1996. "Smoking and Age-Related Maculopathy: The Blue Mountains Eye Study." *Archives of Ophthalmology* 114:1518–1523.

Vingerling, J. R., A. Hofman, D. E. Grobbee et al. 1996. "Age-Related Macular Degeneration and Smoking: The Rotterdam Study." *Archives of Ophthalmology* 114:1193–1196.

West, S., B. Munoz, E. A. Emmett et al. 1989. "Cigarette Smoking and Risk of Nuclear Cataract." *Archives of Ophthalmology* 107:1166–1169.

HIGH-FAT DIET

Mares-Perlman, J. A., W. E. Brady, R. Klein et al. 1955. "Dietary Fat and Age-Related Maculopathy." *Archives of Ophthalmology* 113:743–748.

Sanders, T.A.B., A. P. Haines, R. Wormald et al. 1993. "Essential Fatty Acids, Plasma Cholesterol, and Fat-Soluble Vitamins in Subjects with Age-Related Maculopathy and Matched Control Subjects." *American Journal of Nutrition* 57:428–433.

Vingerling, J. R., I. Dielemans, A. Hofman, et al. 1955. "Age-Related Macular Degeneration Is Associated with Atherosclerosis—The Rotterdam Study." *American Journal of Epidemiology* 142:404–409.

UNPROTECTED EXPOSURE TO SUNLIGHT

Cruickshanks, K. J., R. Klein, and B. E. K. Klein. 1993. "Sunlight and Age-Related Macular Degeneration: The Beaver Dam Eye Study." *Archives of Ophthalmology* 111:514–518.

Ham, W. T., H. A. Mueller, J. J. Ruffolo et al. 1979. "Sensitivity of the Retina to Radiation Damage as a Function of Wavelength." *Photochemistry and Photobiology* 29:735–743.

Ham, W. T., H. A. Mueller, J. J. Ruffolo et al. 1982. "Action Spectrum for Retinal Injury from Near-Ultraviolet Radiation in the Aphakic Monkey." *American Journal of Ophthalmology* 93:299–306.

Harlan, J. B., D. T. Weidenthal, and W. R. Green. 1997. "Histologic Study of a Shielded Macula." *Retina* 17:232–238.

Hecht, S., C. D. Hendley, S. Ross et al. 1948. "The Effect of Exposure to Sunlight on Night Vision." *American Journal of Ophthalmology* 31:1573–1580.

Lawwill, T. 1982. "Three Major Pathologic Processes Caused by Light in the Primate Retina: A Search for Mechanisms." *Transactions American Ophthalmological Society* 80:517–579.

Mainster, M. A. 1987. "Light and Macular Degeneration: A Biophysical and Clinical Perspective." *Eye* 1:304–310.

Noell, W. K. 1980. "Possible Mechanism of Photoreceptor Damage by Light in Mammalian Eyes." *Vision Research* 20:1163–1171.

Ron, S., and J. J. Weiter. 1994. "Light Damage to the Eye." *Journal of the Florida Medical Association* 81:248–251.

Taylor, H. R., S. West, B. Munoz et al. 1992. "The Long-Term Effects of Visible Light on the Eye." *Archives of Ophthalmology* 110:99–104.

West, S. K., F. S. Rosenthal, N. M. Bressler et al. 1989. "Exposure to Sunlight and Other Risk Factors for Age-Related Macular Degeneration." *Archives of Ophthalmology* 107:875–879.

Yannuzzi, L. A., Y. L. Fisher, J. S. Slakter et al. 1989. "Solar Retinopathy: A Photobiologic and Geophysical Analysis." *Retina* 9:28–43.

Young, R. W. 1988. "Solar Radiation and Age-Related Macular Degeneration." *Survey of Ophthalmology* 32:252–269.

HEREDITY

Allikmets, R., N. F. Shroyer, Nanda Singh et al. 1997. "Mutation of the Stargardt Disease Gene (ABCR) in Age-Related Macular Degeneration." *Science* 277:1805–1807.

Meyers, S. M., T. Greene, and F. A. Gutman. 1995. "A Twin Study of Age-Related Macular Degeneration." *American Journal of Ophthalmology* 120:757–66.

Piguet, B., J. A. Wells, I. B. Palmvang et al. 1993. "Age-Related Bruch's Membrane Change: A Clinical Study of the Relative Role of Heredity and Environment." *British Journal of Ophthalmology* 77:400–403.

Silvestri, G., P. B. Johnston, and A. E. Hughes. 1994. "Is Genetic Predisposition an Important Risk Factor in Age-Related Macular Degeneration?" *Eye* 8:564–568.

Zhang, K., T. H. Nguyen, A. Crandal et al. 1955. "Genetic and Molecular Studies of Macular Dystrophies: Recent Developments." *Survey of Ophthalmology* 40:51–61.

RACE AND IRIS COLOR

Schachat, A. P., L. Hyman, C. Leske et al. 1995. "Features of Age-Related Macular Degeneration in a Black Population." *Archives of Ophthalmology* 113:728–735.

GENDER

Smith, W., B. Math, B. Med et al. 1997. "Gender, Oestrogen, Hormone Replacement and Age-Related Macular Degeneration: Results from the Blue Mountains Eye Study." *Australian and New Zealand Journal of Ophthalmology* 25, supplement 1:S13–15.

Chapter 4: Vision and Nutrition: What You Eat Is How You See

Hercberg, S., et al. 1994. *International Journal for Vitamin and Nutrition Research* 64, no. 3:220–232.

Leske, M. C., L. T. Chylack, S. Y. Wu et al. 1991. "The Lens Opacities Case-Control Study. Risk Factors for Cataracts." *Archives of Ophthalmology* 109:244–251.

Mares-Perlman, J. A., B. E. K. Klein, R. Klein et al. 1994. "Relationship Between Lens Opacities and Vitamin and Mineral Supplementation." *Ophthalmology* 101:315–325.

Mares-Perlman, J. A., W. E. Brady, B. E. K. Klein et al. 1995. "Diet and Nuclear Lens Opacities." *American Journal of Epidemiology* 141:322–334.

Newsome, D. A. et al. 1988. "Oral Zinc in Macular Degeneration." *Archives of Ophthalmology* 106:192–198.

Pennington, J. A. T., B. E. Young, D. B. Wilson et al. 1986. "Mineral Content of Foods and Total Diets: The Selected Minerals in Foods Survey 1982–1984." *Journal of the American Dietetic Association* 86:876–878.

Robertson, J. M., A. P. Donner, and J. R. Trevithick. 1991. "A Possible Role for Vitamins C and E in Cataract Prevention." *American Journal of Clinical Nutrition* 53:346S–351S.

Sperduto, R. D., T. S. Hu, R. C. Milton et al. 1993. "The Linxian Cataract Studies: Two Interventional Trials." *Archives of Ophthalmology* 111:1246–1253.

Seddon, J. M., U. A. Ajani, R. D. Sperduto et al. 1994. "Dietary Carotenoids, Vitamin A, C and E, and Advanced Age-Related Macular Degeneration." *Journal of the American Medical Association* 272:1413–1420.

Vitale, S., S. West, J. Hallfrisch et al. 1993. "Plasma Antioxidants and Risk of Cortical and Nuclear Cataracts." *Epidemiology* 4:195–203.

Chapter 5: The Light in Your Eyes

Bergmanson, J. P. G., and P. G. Soderberg. 1998. "The Significance of Ultraviolet Radiation for Eye Diseases." *Dispensing Ophthalmologist UV Compendium*, supplement: 24–33.

Bochow, T. W., S. K. West, A. Azar et al. 1989. "Ultraviolet Light Exposure and Risk of Posterior Subcapsular Cataracts." *Archives of Ophthalmology* 107:369–372.

Brilliant, L. B., N. C. Grasset, R. P. Pokhrel et al. 1983. "Associations Among Cataract Prevalence, Sunlight Hours, and Altitude in the Himalayas." *American Journal of Epidemiology* 118:250–264.

Ham, W. T., H. A. Mueller, J. J. Ruffolo et al. 1979. "Sensitivity of the Retina to Radiation Damage as a Function of Wavelength." *Photochemistry and Photobiology* 29:735–743.

Ham, W. T., H. A. Mueller, J. J. Ruffolo et al. 1982. "Action Spectrum for Retinal Injury from Near-Ultraviolet Radiation in the Aphakic Monkey." *American Journal of Ophthalmology* 93:299–306.

Harlan, J. B., D. T. Weidenthal, and W. R. Green. 1997. "Histologic Study of a Shielded Macula." *Retina* 17:232–238.

Hiller, R., R. D. Sperduto, and F. Ederer. 1986. "Epidemiologic Associations with Nuclear, Cortical, and Posterior Subcapsular Cataracts." *American Journal of Epidemiology* 124:916–925.

Kerr, J. B., and C. T. McElroy. 1998. "Evidence for Large Upward Trends of Ultraviolet-B Radiation Linked to Ozone Depletion." *Dispensing Ophthalmologist UV Compendium suppliment.* 13–16.

Klein, B. E. K., K. J. Cruickshanks, and R. Klein. 1995. "Leisure Time, Sunlight Exposure and Cataracts." *Documenta Ophthalmologica* 88:295–305.

Lawwill, T. 1982. "Three Major Pathologic Processes Caused by Light in the Primate Retina: A Search for Mechanisms." *Transactions of the American Ophthalmologic Society.* 80:517–579.

Mainster, M. A. 1987. "Light and Macular Degeneration: A Biophysical and Clinical Perspective." *Eye* 1:304–310.

Noell, W. K. 1980. "Possible Mechanism of Photoreceptor Damage by Light in Mammalian Eyes." *Vision Research* 20:1163–1171.

Olson, C. M. 1989. "Increased Outdoor Recreation, Diminished Ozone Layer Pose Ultraviolet Radiation Threat to Eye." *Journal of the American Medical Association* 261:1102–1103.

Rosmini, R., M. A. Stazi, R. C. Milton et al. 1994. "A Dose-Response Effect Between a Sunlight Index and Age-Related Cataracts." *Epidemiology* 4:266–270.

Sliney, D. H. 1998. "Epidemiological Studies of Sunlight and Cataract: The Critical Factor of Ultraviolet Exposure Geometry." *Dispensing Ophthalmologist UV Compendium*, supplement: 65–74.

Sliney, D. H. 1998. "Ocular Injury Due to Light Toxicity." *Dispensing Ophthalmologist UV Compendium*, supplement: 17–23.

Taylor, H. R., S. K. West, F. S. Rosenthal et al. 1988. "Effect of Ultraviolet Radiation on Cataract Formation." *New England Journal of Medicine* 319:1429–1433.

Taylor, H. R., and J. C. Javitt. 1998. "Ocular Protection from Solar Radiation." *Duane's Clinical Ophthalmology.* Vol. 5, no. 55. A. E. Jaeger, ed. Philadelphia: Harper & Row. 1–29.

Zuclich, J. A. 1989. "Ultraviolet-Induced Photochemical Damage in Ocular Tissues." *Health Physics* 56:671–682.

Chapter 6: Guidelines for Taking Vitamin and Mineral Supplements

Age-Related Macular Degeneration Study Group. 1996. "Multicenter Ophthalmic and Nutritional Age-Related Macular Degeneration Study, Part 2: Antioxidant Intervention and Conclusion." *Journal of the American Optometric Association* 67:30–49.

The Alpha-tocopherol, Beta-carotene Cancer Prevention Study Group. 1994. "The Effect of Vitamin E and Beta-carotene on the Incidence of Lung Cancer and Other Cancers in Male Smokers." *New England Journal of Medicine* 330:1029–1035.

Bush, A. I., W. H. Pettingell, G. Multhaup et al. 1994. "Rapid Induction of Alzheimer A Beta Amyloid Formation by Zinc." *Science* 265 no. 5177 (2 Sept.): 1464–1467.

Byers, T., and N. Guerrero. 1995. "Epidemiologic Evidence for Vitamin C and Vitamin E in Cancer Prevention." *American Journal of Clinical Nutrition* 62, supplement: 1385S–1392S.

Costantino, J. P., L. H. Kuller, L. Begg et al. 1988. "Serum Level Changes After Administration of a Pharmacologic Dose of Beta-carotene." *American Journal of Clinical Nutrition* 48:1277–1283.

Garewal, H. 1995. "Antioxidants in Oral Cancer Prevention." *American Journal of Clinical Nutrition* 62, supplement: 1410S–1416S.

Karcioglu, Z. A. 1982. "Zinc in the Eye." *Survey of Ophthalmology* 27, no. 2:114–122.

Manon, J. E., et al. 1993. "Antioxidants and Cardiovascular Disease: A Review." *Journal of the American College of Nutrition* 12:426–432.

Meydani, S. N., et al. 1995. "Antioxidants and Immune Response in Aged Persons: Overview of Present Evidence." *American Journal of Clinical Nutrition* 62, supplement: 1462S–1476S.

Newsome, D. A., M. Swartz, N. C. Leone et al. 1988. "Oral Zinc in Macular Degeneration." *Archives of Ophthalmology* 106:192–198.

Rimm, E. B. et al. 1993. "Vitamin E Consumption and the Risk of Coronary Heart Disease in Men." *New England Journal of Medicine* 328:1450–1456.

Stampfer, M. J., et al. 1993. "Vitamin E Consumption and the Risk of Coronary Heart Disease in Women." *New England Journal of Medicine* 328:1444–1449.

Tyler, Varro E., Ph.D. "The Hones Herbal: A Sensible Guide to the Use of Herbal and Related Remedies." Binghamton, N.Y.: Pharmaceutical Products Press (an imprint of The Haworth Press, Inc.)

Vannas, S., and H. Orma. 1958. "On the Treatment of Arteriosclerotic Chorioretinopathy." *Acta Ophthalmologica* 36:601–612.

Van Poppel, G., and R. A. Goldbohm. 1995. "Epidemiologic Evidence for Beta-carotene and Cancer Prevention." *American Journal of Clinical Nutrition* 62, supplement: 1393S–1402S.

West, S., S. Vitale, J. Hallfrisch et al. 1994. "Are Antioxidants or Supplements Protective for Age-Related Macular Degeneration?" *Archives of Ophthalmology* 112:222–227.

Chapter 7: Eat Right and See the Results; Chapter 8: Vegetables Ranked: Four-Star Antioxidants; Chapter 9: Fruit Ranked: Four-Star Antioxidants; Chapter 10: Sources of Beta Carotene, Lutein, and Zeaxanthin; Chapter 11: Common Food Sources of Vitamin C and Vitamin E; Chapter 12: Common Food Sources of Zinc and Other Minerals

Anderson, Jean, and Elaine Hanna. 1985. *The New Doubleday Cookbook*. New York: Doubleday.

Center for Science in the Public Interest. May 1998. *Nutrition Action Healthletter* 25, no. 4.

Mangels, A. R., J. M. Holden, G. R. Beecher et al. 1993. "Carotenoid Content of Fruits and Vegetables: An Evaluation of Analytic Data." *Journal of the American Dietetic Association* 93:284–296.

Rombauer, Irma, and Marion Rombauer Becker. 1975. *Joy of Cooking*. New York: Simon & Schuster.

Ter Meer, Mary, and Jamie Gates Galeana. 1997. *Vegetarian Cooking for Healthy Living*. Mankato, Minn.: Appletree Press.

Chapter 13: How to Buy, Store, and Prepare Vegetables and Fruit for Maximum Nutrition

Carlson, B. L., and M. H. Tabacchi. 1988. "Loss of Vitamin C in Vegetables During the Food Service Cycle." *Journal of the American Dietetic Association* 88:65–67.

Issa, J., and E. A. Mielke. 1980. "Influence of Certain Citrus Interstocks on Beta-carotene and Lycopene Levels in 10-Year-Old "Redbush" Grapefruit." *Journal of the American Society for Horticultural Science* 105:807–809.

Karmas, E., and Robert S. Harris. 1988. *Nutritional Evaluation of Food Processing*. New York: Van Nostrand Reinhold Company.

Klein, B. P., and A. K. Perry. 1982. "Ascorbic Acid and Vitamin A Activity in Selected Vegetables from Different Geographical Areas of the United States." *Journal of Food Science* 47:941–945.

Kramer, A. 1974. "Storage Retention of Nutrients." *Food Technology*, 50–58.

Krehl, W. A., and R. W. Winters. 1950. "Effect of Cooking Methods on Retention of Vitamins and Minerals in Vegetables." *Journal of the American Dietetic Association* 26:966–972.

Noble, I., and J. Worthington. 1948. "Ascorbic Acid Retention in Cooked Vegetables." *Journal of Home Economics* 129–130.

Pantastico, E. B., and O. Bautista. 1976. "Post-Harvest Handling of Tropical Vegetable Crops." *Horticultural Science* 11:122–124.

Russell, L. F., W. J. Mullin, and D. F. Wood. 1983. "Vitamin C Content of Fresh Spinach." *Nutritional Reports International* 5:1149–1158.

Sweeney, J. P., and A. C. Marsh. 1971. "Effect of Processing on Provitamin A in Vegetables." *Journal of the American Dietetic Association* 59:238–242.

Thompson, D. R. 1982. "The Challenge in Predicting Nutrient Changes During Food Processing." *Food Technology* 97–115.

Van den Berg, L., and C. P. Lentz. 1978. "High Humidity Storage of Vegetables and Fruits." *Horticultural Science* 13:565–569.

Chapter 16: Cultivate a Healthy Lifestyle Without Tobacco or Alcohol

Obisesan, T. O., R. Hirsch, O. Kosoko et al. 1998. "Moderate Wine Consumption Is Associated with Decreased Odds of Developing Age-Related Macular Degeneration in NHANES-1." *Journal of American Geriatric Science* 46:1–7.

See also references for chapter 3.

Chapter 17: Choose the Right Sunglasses

Clark, B., et al. 1946. "The Effect of Sunlight on Dark Adaptation." *American Journal of Ophthalmology* 29:828.

Cruickshanks, K. J., R. Klein, and B. E. K. Klein. 1993. "The Beaver Dam Eye Study: Sunlight and Age-Related Macular Degeneration." *Archives of Ophthalmology* 111:514–518.

Ham, W. T., et al. 1979. "Sensitivity of the Retina to Radiation Damage as a Function of Wavelength." *Photochemistry and Photobiology* 29:735–743.

Hecht, S., et al. 1948. "The Effect of Exposure to Sunlight on Night Vision." *American Journal of Ophthalmology* 31:1573.

MacDonald, P. R. 1949. "Evaluation of Night Vision." *American Journal of Ophthalmology* 32:1535.

Magnante, D. O. B., and D. Miller. 1985. "Ultraviolet Absorption of Commonly Used Clip-On Sunglasses." *Annals of Ophthalmology* 17:614–616.

Peckham, R. H. 1947. "The Protection and Maintenance of Night Vision for Military Personnel." *American Journal of Ophthalmology* 30:1588.

Peckham, R. H., and R. D. Harley. 1951. "The Effect of Sunglasses in Protecting Retinal Sensitivity." *American Journal of Ophthalmology* 34:1499–1507.

Rosenthal, F. S., et al. 1988. "The Effect of Sunglasses on Ocular Exposure to Ultraviolet Radiation." *American Journal of Public Health* 78:72–74.

Taylor, H. R., and J. C. Javitt. 1988. "Ocular Protection from Solar Radiation." *Duane's Clinical Ophthalmology.* Vol. 5, no. 55. A. E. Jaeger, ed. Philadelphia: Harper & Row. 1–29.

Werner, J. S. 1991. "Children's Sunglasses: Caveat Emptor." *Optometry & Vision Science* 68:318–320.

See also references for chapter 3.

Part Three: Recipes to Prevent Macular Degeneration

First Data Bank, Inc. 1998. "Nutritionist Five." San Bruno, Calif.: The Hearst Corporation.

Mangels, A. R., J. M. Holden, G. R. Becher et al. 1993. "Carotenoid Content of Fruits and Vegetables: An Evaluation of Analytic Data." *Journal of the American Dietetic Association* 93:284–296.

Index

About the Author

Alexander M. Eaton, M.D., graduated magna cum laude from Duke University, then attended Duke University Medical School and completed a residency at Columbia University–Presbyterian Medical Center in New York. After completing his formal training, Dr. Eaton returned to Duke University to join the faculty, and was named Chief Resident. He completed a Retina Fellowship at Duke University before leaving to join Eye Centers of Florida.

Dr. Eaton, a Diplomate of the American Board of Ophthalmology, is a pioneer in the use of the laser, and is the inventor of numerous laser-activated medical devices. As the author of more than fifteen published professional papers, his significant contributions to medicine have been featured in *The New York Times.* He serves as an assistant professor at the University of South Florida, teaching and conducting research, and as a consulting research associate at Duke University, where he collaborates with Duke's biophysics laboratory on the development and modification of instruments for ocular surgery. He is also active in FDA studies evaluating new treatments for macular degeneration: one on the use of photodynamic therapy (PDT) for wet macular degeneration, and the other on RheoTherapy for dry macular degeneration.

Dr. Eaton currently practices medicine in Fort Myers, Florida, and is head of the Retina Department at Eye Centers of Florida, a progressive ophthalmology practice with six physicians, twenty-three optometrists, and a staff of more than three hundred in twenty offices throughout Southwest Florida.

Other Members of the Team

Chef Eric Truglas is an award-winning chef who is listed in *Top 2,000 Chefs of America.* A graduate of the Lycée d'État D'Hôtellerie in France and a member of the World Master Chef Society, Chef Truglas is the author of a gourmet cookbook, *Cuisine du Soleil.* He is often invited to present culinary classes to corporate and other groups, and makes frequent guest appearances on national television, including the Discovery Channel and Fit TV. Chef Truglas's experience includes service as executive chef at Sanibel Harbour Resort and Spa, Florida, at the Meridien Hotel in Boston, and as a restaurant owner.

Chef Todd Johnson has also won awards for nutritious meals that are both interesting and appealing. He is a graduate of Johnson & Wales University, Miami, and holds an Associate of Science degree in culinary arts. His experience includes working with Mark Militello, chef/owner of Mark's Place in Miami. He has served as executive sous-chef at Chef's Garden Restaurant in Naples, Florida (which earned *Florida Trend* magazine's Golden Spoon Award as one of the top twenty restaurants in Florida), and at other award-winning establishments in Southwest Florida.

Chef Joy Purcell is a graduate of the Culinary Institute of America, New York, and is certified in nutritional cooking and cuisine. In addition to her regular duties as catering chef at one of Southwest Florida's leading heart institutes, Chef Purcell is sole owner of Creations, a custom catering business.

Jamie Gates Galeana, M.S., R.D., L.D., holds a Master of Science degree in nutrition from Boston University and a Bachelor of Science degree in dietetics and nutrition from Florida International University, Miami. She specializes in cardiovascular, wellness, and sports nutrition.

Ms. Galeana, a recognized public speaker and freelance writer, is coauthor of *Vegetarian Cooking for Healthy Living*, which received the Benjamin Franklin Gold Star Award for Best New Voice of 1998, and was selected as one of the Top 10 Health and Fitness Books of 1997 by the *University of Texas Lifetime Health Letter.* She assisted with the preparation of the chapters on diet, vegetables and fruits, and recipes.

Ginger Patterson, Ph.D., R.D., L.D, performed the nutritional analysis for the recipe section, and reviewed the sections on nutrition. She holds a master's degree in adult education and a bachelor's degree in human nutrition from Rutgers University. Dr. Patterson also earned a second master's degree and her doctorate in psychology from California Coast University.

An adjunct professor of nutrition at Florida Gulf Coast University, Dr. Patterson is a frequent speaker on dietary and fitness topics throughout the United States, and writes for magazines and appears on regional television programs. She also serves as nutrition supervisor at the Wellness Center of Lee Memorial Hospital in Fort Myers, Florida.